Thank You God for Cancer

By

Michael E LaRiviere

and

Judy LaRiviere

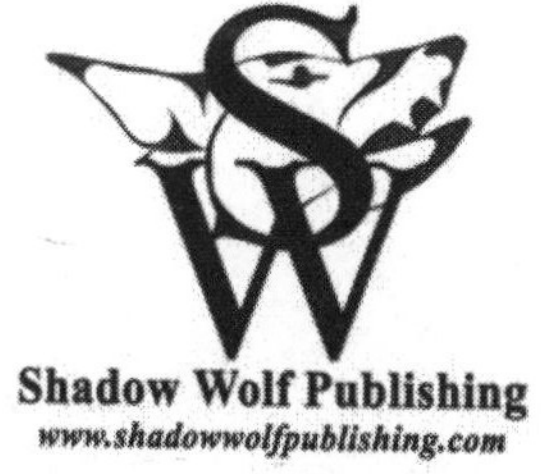

Thank You God for Cancer

Introduction by

Doctor John Finley

Special thanks to friends who allowed their stories to be told:

Cover Art by

D E LaRiviere and Donna LaRiviere

Photography by

D E LaRiviere

Editor
Judy LaRiviere

Special contributors who made this book possible:

Helen Steiner Rice, Lynn Eib, Reverend Sharon Herlihy, Gigi Lee Pastor Jeff Hardy, Doctor Stan and Carol Crunk, West Cancer Treatment Clinic, American Cancer Society, Wings Cancer Foundation, Faye Russell, Sheila Harrell, Charles Biggs, Vicky Evans, Walter and Martha Edwards, our Branson, Missouri friends Ray and Sonia Tucker and Paul, Annette and Nicole Yendez

For information on other books from Shadow Wolf Publishing
Please visit our website at

www.shadowwolfpublishing.com

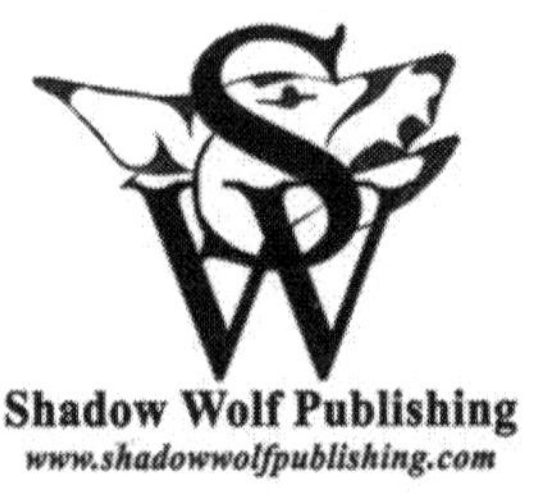

Prologue

The focus of this book is patients who have been diagnosed with one or more of the numerous kinds of cancer that plague humanity and who have joined a unique family which inhabits the oftentimes dark, fearful, and unsettling world that is unlike any other world.

The target audience for this book is simple yet very large. It is comprised of patients, care givers, medical and administrative professionals, researchers, and two groups of precious people that we will call victims and survivors or overcomers. These groups are broken down into two groups: believers in the God of the Bible, and those who do not embrace these beliefs.

To the former group we endeavor to bring comfort, encouragement, strength, and Scriptural insights. To the latter, we try our best to present the Gospel in such a way as to help them to appreciate the Christian world and perhaps accept Jesus Christ as their Lord and Savior.

Our motivation lies in the time tested and proven truths that when Jesus enters the life of a believer, He brings with Him a myriad of blessings, promises, strengths, and victories. He bids his children to rest in, rely upon, and submit to those powerful benefits of a relationship with Him. We know of no greater comfort than Jesus Christ amid the discomforts of cancer.

Friedrich Nietzsché once said, “That which does not kill us makes us stronger.” Although oftentimes this may be a true statement, it is not always so. We have observed the lives of cancer patients change for the better as well as for the worse. Peace, patience, and perseverance on the one hand can likewise turn to bitterness, blame, and an angry negative spirit that makes life miserable for both the care recipient and the care giver.

We have witnessed miraculous healings and abject failures of the best medical efforts applied to the same types of cancer but in uniquely different patients. We learn that doctors practice medicine, but only God grants the healing.

We have prayed with people who suffer a great deal from the treatments, some whose life is maintained and prolonged through the treatments but experience significant discomfort through it all.

So what about the precious promises in Scripture that seem to say one thing but produce something quite different than expected? Cancer treatment requires hard work, extreme patience, a positive frame of mind, and a deep faith in God.

Sometimes a cure for cancer comes only in Heaven and for care-givers that adds mourning and grief to the long list of sacrifices and discomforts experienced by loved ones who must watch the challenges of a very sick, weak, confused, fearful patient.

This book tells the heartfelt stories of those whose lives have been changed by the cancer experience and have joined a throng of believers who can stand up and praise God for their spiritual growth and say in unison, "Thank you God for Cancer."

We'll finish this prologue by sharing a passage of Scripture from the book of Luke Chapter 9 and verse 23 in the New International Version. *"Then he said to them all: "Whoever wants to be my disciple must deny themselves and take up their cross daily and follow me."*

The Christian cancer patient will share in Christ's suffering and death by taking up his or her cross and offering the pain and discomfort of the disease in memoriam to His sacrifice.

On the other hand, some may cast railing accusations against God for allowing the cancer in the first place. Cancer is not the cross that we must take up and bear –it's the pain and possible death that it brings and the oftentimes nearly unbearable demands on the patient and loved ones.

God bless you as you read this work. If you should ever need us, you know where to find us.

§§§

This book is dedicated to the memory of

Our niece and great-niece

Cheryl Knight Wilson

and

Shannon Wilson-Harness

Mother and Daughter

Died to this world and to cancer; Alive and safe in the arms of Jesus

A Work In Progress

This book is called a work in progress because the characters and incidents are real as well as the truths that are presented. Every person that we mention is a work in progress. They will be such until their time on earth is finished and we are all called home to have our personal work in progress reviewed.

The Supreme Judge will determine the degree to which we have successfully grown in His image and what we did with what He gave us.

Some thoughts and life lessons are based on truth as Judy and I understand it and have applied to our own lives. So like this book, we too are a work in progress and far from finished.

We live in a time of unparalleled stress on both the young and old. Drug and alcohol abuse is rampant and the movement away from God in our country is alarming.

Statistics from reliable reporting agencies indicate that about 50% of all human beings on this planet already have or will contract cancer in their lifetime and those figures are increasing every year.

The jobless rate is increasing, our national debt is out of control, and the nuclear family is collapsing all around us.

The national morale is very low and trust in government is nearly non-existent. Loyalty within the workplace, spiritual leadership in the home, decency, morality, purity, virginity, righteousness, and holiness are waning concepts.

Is there anything still true, still strong enough to change lives for the better, intervene in hopelessness, and provide vision to a blind world? Yes there is.

His name is Jesus, His instructions can be found in the Bible, His promises are true, and His mercy, grace, and forgiveness are free for the asking.

As we trek through the thorn and thistle laden pathways of cancer, we always find what Judy and I call *God Things*. They belong only to God; only He knows the reasons behind them, and sometimes He just does not explain them to mere humans. That's what makes them *God Things*.

God Bless you and be merciful to you in this journey of challenge, victory, defeat, and sharing with others of your cancer family.

§§§

Introduction

"Cancer" is one of the most frightening words in the English language. Add the words "you have" to the sentence, and even the strongest person will want to go to their knees, in fear or in prayer. Even with all the new technologies, treatments and advancements, people still suffer . . . and die with cancer.

I am the pastor of Bartlett Hills Baptist Church. I love being their pastor. With all of the joy that I experience here, I know that being the shepherd means I will walk with my people in some of their hardest times and darkest hours.

As pastors, we always struggle with how to best minister to people in need. We desire to show God's love and grace, to encourage and pray, and to see God work in all circumstances. **God has moved in our congregation in recent days to take us to a place of new insight and ministry.** That is how this book came to be.

In mid-July of 2013, I preached a Sunday morning sermon that God had placed on my heart. Little did I realize that focus of the message would have such swift and dramatic impact on several lives in our church.

"No matter what the circumstance . . . major illness, catastrophe, loss of a family member, reversal of fortune or

any other tragedy . . . trust Jesus." Obvious truth, yet often, hard to live out.

During a reception that evening, one of our faithful members approached me to express how the sermon touched him. He had received an unsettling report from his doctor confirming that he had cancer. I could hear the stress in his voice as he asked for prayer.

This man has a strong teaching ministry. Where his cancer was located could possibly impact or end that ministry. It would be "life changing."

What really brought the sermon home to me personally was that in just over a week, I was in the hospital recovering from triple by-pass surgery that was totally unexpected.

I am an avid runner, tennis player and advocate of good health. I was reminded that we can't change our health history and we can't stop ailments and illnesses.

During that same period of time, others in our church suffered from cancer and other health problems. **Life goes on . . . will we trust Jesus?** What does "trusting Jesus?" look like in real life? How does God use our experiences to prepare us for an even greater opportunity to minister to and encourage others?

The member who approached me suffered a great deal for a long time – over eight months. He lost a significant amount of weight, hair, muscle tone, and was immobile on an increasing scale with each treatment of chemo-therapy.

I must say, he and his lovely wife are different people today in a most positive way. Their testimony and trust in Jesus are priceless and they are an encouragement to any who hear them.

These events and those of the past have reinforced the need (and opportunity) to provide help to hurting souls. Based upon personal need in our church and the potential for giving God glory, our church body has launched a vital ministry in the form of a **cancer support group.**

Mike and Judy LaRiviere have co-written this book entitled "Thank you God for Cancer." An emphasis has been placed on the proper interpretation of Scripture and personal relationship with Jesus so that even in times of great stress, depression, and need for encouragement, our people can depend upon the precious promises of the loving kindness of God that never stops but endures forever.

Jesus loves us unconditionally; we live and have our being in Him; and everything He is, we are. There is so much potential power and peace in that truth.

I am excited about the future of this ministry, and I'm happy that our church is taking a leadership role in cancer support in league with the West Cancer Clinic based WINGS Cancer Foundation.

Sharon Herlihy, Chaplain, West Clinic WINGS Foundation is providing guidance and support to this ministry, and we appreciate her efforts in our behalf.

John Finley, Pastor
Bartlett Hills Baptist Church

§§§

Most Common Cancer Types

This list of common cancer types includes those that are diagnosed with the greatest frequency in the United States, excluding non-melanoma skin cancers:

- Bladder
- Breast
- Colon and Rectal
- Endometrial
- Kidney
- Leukemia
- Lung
- Melanoma
- Non-Hodgkin Lymphoma
- Pancreatic
- Prostate
- Thyroid

Cancer incidence and mortality statistics reported by the American Cancer Society and other resources were used to create the above list and is provided for general information purposes only.

§§§

Chapter One

The Beginning and the End

How do we begin a book about the highs and lows of the human experience? About ultimate fears realized, and the greatest of disappointments. This book is about being out of control, and where the treatment for a disease is often more devastating than is the disease itself. It depicts the ending of one life and style and the beginning of another. It also means saying goodbye to what has been significant in life, and then searching for a new significance.

To begin, we have found a poem that aptly describes how our life's journey can take a significant change in direction, and how, if left to our own strength and devices, that change of direction could have destroyed us. But God has a plan for our lives, and He is sovereign, loving, and good –He is also in control.

Helen Steiner Rice (May 19, 1900 – April 23, 1981) was a writer of religious and inspirational poetry. She has been acclaimed as America's beloved inspirational poet laureate. Her Christian faith and penning skills, in concert with her ability to express deep emotion have rendered her works immortal. One poem stands out among the others as fitting to this book. A Bend in the Road is most famous and beloved by countless people seeking beauty among the ashes and solace for their hurting hearts.

Thank You God for Cancer

When we feel we have nothing left to give
And we are sure that the song has ended
When our day seems over and the shadows fall
And the darkness of night has descended.

Where can we go to find the strength
To valiantly keep on trying,
Where can we find the hand that will dry
The tears that the heart is crying.

There's but one place to go and that is to God
And dropping all pretense and pride,
We can pour out our problems without restraint
And gain strength from Him at our side.

And together we stand at life's crossroads
And view what we think is the end
But God has a much bigger vision
And He tells us it's only a bend.

For the road goes on and is smoother
And the pause in the song is a rest
And the part that's unsung and unfinished
Is the sweetest and richest and best.

So rest and relax and grow stronger
Let go and let God share your load
Your work is not finished or ended,
You've just come to a bend in the road.

§

Judy and I have been married for over fifty years; have two sons, who are married to wonderful ladies, and two beautiful granddaughters. We have managed and retired from three careers and are now experiencing what many might call the good life.

We are members of a strong and loving church and have an unshakable Christian faith. We have everything good that this world has to offer. We are also both cancer survivors.

My beloved and I have gone through the terrors, pain, frustrations, fears, apprehensions, and insecurities that often come with the cellular abnormality disease called cancer.

Judy has had endometrial and colon cancer about a decade apart. I contracted Squamous cell carcinoma a year before beginning this book.

Interestingly, I was the care giver for Judy as she went through her personal ordeals, and then we changed roles and she became my caregiver. We both have experience in giving and receiving care and the frustrations involved in both.

I find no better phrase to describe what Judy and I went through in our journey toward spiritual maturity and physical healing than was coined by sixteenth century, Saint John of the Cross.

Saint John wrote about the journey of the soul toward union with God. He called it "the dark night", representing the hardships and difficulties a soul encounters in detachment from this world and reaching the light of the union with the Creator in the next.

The Dark Night of the Soul reflects painful experiences endured in seeking to grow to spiritual maturity and a closer relationship with God. That is so fitting here.

Somewhere along the treacherous path of our dark night, Judy and I lost much of our dignity, identity, confidence, self assuredness; and our modesty was seriously injured on more than one occasion.

Then, somewhere a little farther down that path, we recovered the more important things, and we both found from where our real help and strength came.

We wrote this book so that others might identify with us and realize that they are not alone in their fight, and they are not the only ones in the world that have experienced the many challenges of what may be the most frightening word in our vocabulary – *Cancer.*

§

Our journey through this dark and often frightening world of ominous things and foreboding experiences began unexpectedly, continued uncontrollably, punished us unmercifully, but culminated in our becoming cancer survivors able to lift our hands toward heaven and say in unison, "Thank you God for Cancer."

Now before you pass judgment and suspect that we have lost it, let us explain what we mean. Let us tell you our stories and the stories of some of our friends who can say with us that they are better people for having fought cancer and won the battle.

We are going to share with you learned truths, mistakes, suggestions, and scriptural insights that made a tremendous difference in our lives.

This book is meant to be neither ugly nor pretty, but lays bare the facts that surround being a cancer patient or survivor as we are now called within the circles of the experts.

Please realize that not all cancer patients that avail themselves of chemotherapy, surgery, radiation, and other forms of treatment will experience what we went through, just like we did. These are our stories and do not reflect the way that others might experience the side effects of any of them.

Don't let this book frighten you, and read on past the beginning and through the entire book to see how it all ends before making any judgment calls on treatments, processes, etc.

Allow me to preface the hardships with a major breakthrough for us that came when we found that oftentimes the most fitting prayers are those that do not follow some kind of rule for talking with God.

Judy and I found that oftentimes our heartfelt prayers were not very polished, often were wrapped in panic, always choked out in abject need, and sometimes blurted out at the end of our rope. No matter the delivery, we knew in our spirits that our petitions were heard by a loving God.

This is a great opportunity to introduce you to something we learned from Scripture, which became very real and comforting to us. We call it the Abba, Father, Daddy prayer. Abba is a New Testament Aramaic word that Jesus used for his heavenly father in the most intimate sense.

In *Galatians 4:6*, the apostle Paul wrote, *Because you are his sons, God sent the Spirit of His Son into our hearts, the Spirit who calls out, "Abba, Father".*

We have been given access to the Father in the same intimate and loving way that Jesus approached him. I promise you that there will be times when no other prayer will work. As an example, one night in the hospital, I was crashing under the continual bad news and really scary treatment mandates.

Praying to Lord Jesus or King Jesus just didn't seem right; I needed my Abba at that point, not my brother or Lord or Master. I remember breaking down and praying –no *crying*, "Daddy, your child is losing it, I need you."

Try to remember this when you face the deep blackness of darkness of your dark night of the soul.

§

Mike. I would like to begin with a synopsis or overview of what it was like for me and my physiology to experience chemo therapy.

Others can expect in varying degrees to go through like situations if they should find themselves in the infusion room of a cancer treatment clinic, or a hospital bed with the chemicals being introduced by IV into a vein. IV is the abbreviation for *intravenous*. We will elaborate on the details as the book unfolds.

Please also note that I was given three of the strongest chemo's all in one treatment with each infusion session several weeks apart. There are several different chemo's and each does something different than the others and has its own side effects.

Also, each infusion builds on the last and they become stronger en-masse.

My last chemo infusion was in January 2013. It took about four months to recover from the five treatments that began after I was diagnosed in August 2013. The blisters, bad taste, yeast infection, and gum discomfort known as *thrush*, were probably the least of my woes. In fact, the medicated magical mouthwash to combat it was worse than the mouth sores.

This ravishing and sometimes unmerciful process totally consumed me, and after treatment four, left me mostly helpless, powerless, devoid of good *eustress* and in its place filled my waning body with a cruel and unrelentingly bad *distress*.

On two occasions I felt myself actually slipping out of life and dying, and were it not for hospital intervention, I believe I would have.

The stress was unbelievable at times. Yet I had no emotional strength to fight it. The whole time, I felt Jesus' presence, and it was like when I was a child, my mother used to just be with me during my bouts with nausea and dizziness. I was just as sick, but there was something about her being there….

In reflection, the last nine months of treatment and recovery were indescribably difficult to handle for both Judy and me. Obviously, since I am helping to write this book, I made it through and came out on the other side.

I found myself wracked with weakness, nauseated by the thought of real food, dehydrated to the point of delirium, with the wasting away caused by starvation and all its attachments.

Often I lay motionless as tears ran down my face and I contemplated the death process. Sometimes I just wanted to die and go on to Heaven.

I became like a Weeble, wobbling across the room, bumping onto walls and clutching the kitchen island, refrigerator, or bedstead for balance. Unlike the famous Weeble toy, I did often fall down.

Periodically I would view myself in the bathroom mirror as a bald skeleton, whose rib cage was very pronounced on a body without hair anywhere, except my eyebrows that never completely fell out.

That sounds like a silly little thing, but unless you have experienced it, you can't know the comfort that just having eyebrows can bring to a bald skeleton.

Food of any kind was repulsive and I survived on two protein drinks a day for seven months. That prompted a weight loss of 130 pounds while inactivity prompted the atrophy and subsequent disappearance of most all my muscles.

For some unknown psychological reason, I watched cooking shows that in some way helped me get through my loss of appetite. I would watch steaks, and BBQ, chicken and fish being prepared and served, and for some reason, I placed myself in the picture –get the picture?

By the way, I failed to say that in preparation for radiation, all my teeth except the six in front, top and bottom were pulled. Too late, I opted out of radiation, and now I am paying the price of not having grinder teeth. I often look a bit like a squirrel nibbling at food with his front teeth. My granddaughters get a kick out of it.

We joke about "chemo brain," but I couldn't remember anything from one moment to the next. I forgot common words. I didn't care about anything; I came to hate all the water I had to drink; and actually kind of looked forward to my next protein drink.

The extent of my life for nine months was lying in a recliner or bed; laboring to get to and from the bathroom to urinate; and being painfully constipated and often impacted without a bowel movement for up to ten days. Extreme stomach cramps were frequent. Sorry if that seems a bit too graphic, but try being there.

I am on the other side now of the chemo woes, but I am now dealing with the aftermath of surgery that removed the residual tissue from the tumor in my sinus cavity.

§

I do now have hair, am able once again to walk, and can no longer pull out the old cancer card to get out of housework.

Never make light of chemo or radiation. Everyone is different and can expect different things, but mostly everyone can expect some things, and that is what this book is all about.

Chemotherapy, like radiation, is brutal. I passed out several times, fell often, saw the proverbial light at the end of the tunnel several times as the hot water from the shower bombarded my bald head, and was weakened so much in the shower I would just pass out. Placing a plastic yard chair in the shower as a seat helped with the fainting.

We made trip after trip to the hospital. I remember once urinating all over myself as I passed out and making the ambulance trip in urine saturated clothes on a very chilly night.

How I remember being admitted for a low heart rate (less than thirty and in danger of a heart attack,) loosing whole blood and platelets and my liver and kidneys trying to shut down from the poison. Fluids were administered continuously.

By the way, let me stop here to remember the sweet gift of a loving and caring nurse who early-on gave us her nursing school finger monitor that displays oxygenation and heart rate. That's how we knew I needed help on two occasions. Thank you, precious lady and God bless you.

I think in retrospect, that there were many factors that prompted my full recovery and present freedom from cancer. Each was important; each contributed to the synergy of spiritual and physical wholeness.

I'll not list all of those supporting factors, but our Lord Jesus, my wife Judy, family, friends, doctors, nurses, Ear, Nose and Throat Group, Inc., West Cancer Treatment Center, and the wonderful volunteers of the Wings Foundation, Sunday School class, church family, and the thousands of prayers, cards, visits, and calls all joined to get me where I am today. Oh yes, a precious lady and two dogs get a whole chapter in this book.

Through it all, I maintained gratitude, a positive attitude, and praised God for his mercy and loving kindness. Our electronic social media personal page was a God-send that kept our friends up-to-date. The encouragement we received from our friends was invaluable.

For a while, the dark night of the soul was my constant companion. I watched through dimming eyes as my bride of fifty years wept in anxiety, not being able to fix it.

I didn't mention the tracheotomy that required Judy to clean and maintain the plastic pipe in my throat that was always full of bloody slime –more to come on that also.

This is not the entire bleak picture of most people who undergo chemotherapy. It is simply meant to draw your attention to a situation that unless my Lord and Savior had intervened, I don't think I would have made it. Please read on.

I was so sensitive to the chemotherapy that my oncologist stopped the last treatment in fear that it might kill me. But you know, at that point I didn't care. I would have welcomed death as an escape from the torture of modern medicine and advanced treatments.

I do believe that if chemo had been around for the 12th and 13th century Inquisition, the inquisitors would have used it for torture.

§

We'll call this section simply Endoscopic Sinus Surgery Ethnoidectomy. I'll begin with a fitting quote. "Lord, what fools these mortals be!" These words were spoken by Puck, a mischievous elf in Shakespeare's play A Midsummer Night's Dream written about 1595. Well, they still hold true today.

I opted out of this surgery early on, because what began as one surgeon recommending doing simple micro-surgery to scrape out residual tumor tissue, ended up with a brain surgeon taking over the entire planning process.

His suggestion was to do a craniotomy to make sure he got it all. What would the side effects be from the surgery? Complete loss of smell, possible epilepsy with seizures, anti seizure medication, no driving for six months, and other pleasant things.

In retrospect, I actually thought that the tumor I had in my sinus area was perhaps the size of a grape and that I could dissolve it with salt water over time. None of my doctors explained to me that the actual tumor had filled the left sinus area and that everywhere the tumor had touched might eventually become cancerous again. So the information that I was using to process my decisions was faulty to say the least.

When my ENT, the surgeon, brain surgeon, and my oncologist all began urging me to have the surgery, I began to listen to the experts. The mass had started to grow and brain scans suggested it was becoming vital to have it removed. I gave up and gave in and I am writing this four weeks after the surgery.

I was surprised that the surgery was so extremely invasive and required the attending brain surgeon to scrape and remove a portion of my skull and insert a bridge at the base of the brain to separate it from my sinuses.

The ENT surgeon cleaned everything out with special tools allowing her to remove a mass the size of a chicken egg. The team said that they felt they were able to get everything and I have no scars or visible incision points anywhere. The craniotomy had not been necessary.

When I awoke from the surgery, I had little or no pain, but I had to lie on my back and not move around for seventy-two hours so as not to promote spinal fluid leakage from the brain. That was fun, and I found out just how many places on my body could itch.

For four days in ICU, I ate nothing and drank nothing. I was getting everything from IVs and had no thirst or appetite; I also had no taste or smell. What appeared to be hospital food turned out to be tasteless masses of chewable pulp.

The surgeons were proud of their work as was I. I left the hospital a bit wobbly and dizzy with just a touch of a headache. The only evidence of surgery was a thin thread or wire sticking out of my nose that would prove to be representative of the worst short spurt of discomfort of the whole ordeal.

A few days after my release, I went to the surgeon's office where they removed the packing from my nose by pulling on that string. The packing was the size of my largest finger and just as long. I really thought my brain was being pulled out of my nose.

But I could breathe, and it took about three weeks to get rid of the bloody ooze leavings and pieces of packing. The terrors that I had imagined were just that, imagination.

The mass that the surgeons removed was cancerous and had to be presented to a tumor board. The members of the board make recommendations as to treatment. In the world of cancer, one never knows what the outcome of tests will be until they come back from formal analysis. Mine turned out positive.

I must say that every doctor who treated me in any way has been extremely nice and allayed my fears to the point that I feel rather foolish for ever having doubted them.

Needless to say, I was very foolish for thinking I could just delay the inevitable and not have the surgery. Wishful thinking could have ended in tragedy and the return of my cancer. The experts know what they are doing, what to look for, and what to do about what they find. I do not and I say to little Puck, "yes what a fool *this* mortal be".

§

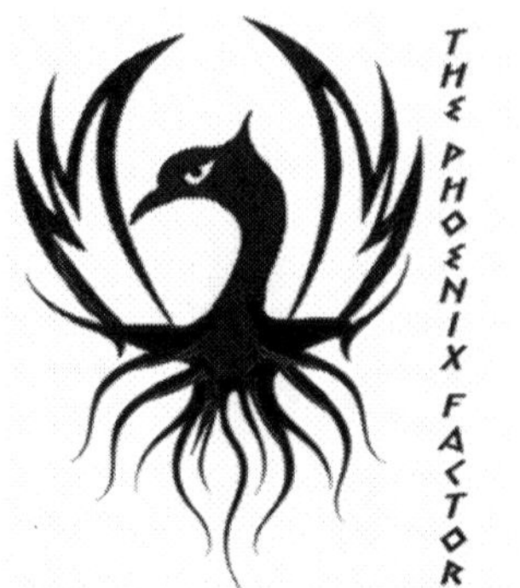

The Phoenix Factor is taken from the mythological bird that was destroyed in flames but rose to begin a new life from the ashes of its original life. We use the Phoenix to introduce the positive changes that can come from the cancer experience.

Our journey was very tough on both Judy and me, but we made it. I want to end this chapter by providing an insight into a favorite passage of Scripture for many people. *Philippians 4:13* says: *"I can do all this through him who gives me strength."*

That wonderfully true passage does not say it will be easy, quick, or a piece of cake. God simply is promising to be with us and to work out his plan for us as we suffer. Just like Jesus suffered. The suffering for Him, we'll call cross-bearing from here on out –not the cancer, but the suffering.

One more vital truth that Judy and I believe is important to those who suffer from cancer or its treatment is that Christianity does not teach continual health, wealth, and prosperity.

§§§

Chapter Two

Judy's Story

Ephesians 6:10-18 (From the Message (MSG))

10-12 .....God is strong, and He wants you strong. So take everything the Master has set out for you, well-made weapons of the best materials. And put them to use so you will be able to stand up to everything the Devil throws your way. This is no afternoon athletic contest that we'll walk away from and forget about in a couple of hours. This is for keeps, a life-or-death fight to the finish against the Devil and all his angels.

13-18 Be prepared. You're up against far more than you can handle on your own. Take all the help you can get, every weapon God has issued, so that when it's all over but the shouting you'll still be on your feet. Truth, righteousness, peace, faith, and salvation are more than words. Learn how to apply them. You'll need them throughout your life. God's Word is an indispensable weapon. In the same way, prayer is essential in this ongoing warfare. Pray hard and long. Pray for your brothers and sisters. Keep your eyes open. Keep each other's spirits up so that no one falls behind or drops out.

§

Judy. The date is August 15, 1996. This is possibly one of the most exciting days of our lives. Our family has gathered together at Baptist Hospital awaiting the birth of our first grandchild.

Scarlett Elizabeth was born at 10:00 p.m. weighing exactly nine pounds. Our son, Darrell became a dad; his wife Donna a mom for the first time. Mike and I and Donna's parents all became first time grandparents. Darrell and Donna both have brothers who became uncles that night. It was a time of rejoicing. Scarlett Elizabeth has brought much joy into all our lives.

Fast forward to August 15, 2013. Scarlett turned 17 years old today. This was possibly the most difficult day of our lives. We learned that her beloved PawPaw Mike has cancer.

How can our worlds be turned upside down so quickly? He hadn't been feeling sick, just had a stuffy nose and sometimes had difficulty swallowing.

Doctors ran several tests that disclosed Mike had two significant tumors; one in the left sinus cavity area and another at the base of his tongue. It seemed surreal; they were telling us he had to have a tracheostomy because of the location and size of the mass on his tongue. If it enlarged due to treatment or surgery, he wouldn't be able to breathe.

How could this be true? He didn't look or act sick. We asked friends to pray, and we began the journey to hell and back. He was told by the doctors that the treatment would be brutal. We had no idea….. Since he has already covered a lot of the details regarding the next few months I won't repeat all of the ways that my beloved suffered.

I was immediately thrown into a very unfamiliar world. After three weeks in the hospital we came home, and I was suddenly responsible for doing things I didn't feel adequate to do.

Much of my day was spent caring for my husband, and a good bit of time was spent on my knees asking God to help me through this demanding and terrifying ordeal.

Mike couldn't eat, so I had to monitor all intake and output. It was so scary. If I didn't clean and care for his trach properly, I could kill him. The word *responsibility* took on a new dimension.

Every evening, close to trach cleaning time and our daily ritual, I asked for direction and strength from the Great Physician. He never failed me or left me on my own to do this task.

When bedtime came I had to get Mike ready and make sure all the equipment was hooked up properly. I'm not a doctor, a nurse, or a respiratory therapist; how was I supposed to do all this? I couldn't, but the Lord guided my hands and my heart during the times when my head didn't know what to do.

In fact, as I think back to it, it wasn't until I prayed and confessed to my inadequacy that God really stepped in and took over. Things seemed to become natural and normal where before they were foreign and incomprehensible.

All of a sudden, my husband of almost fifty years was totally dependent on me. He couldn't eat, so we starved together. Weight began falling off both of us.

I am so thankful for Home Health services. They came weekly and gave us good advice, but at the end of the day it was just the two of us depending on God to get us through the black nights. Some nights were very lonely and dark while others were frightening and demanded more than I had to give.

We went to West Clinic regularly for IV fluids to keep Mike from dehydrating. He drank protein drinks and I ate whatever I could manage to get down. I had to stay on my feet so I could care for him.

One night was particularly scary as he kept getting more incoherent following a treatment. I called the clinic and the doctor on-call called me back immediately.

The doctor said "Go to the emergency room!" I explained that I couldn't get him into the car. He said, "Don't try; call 911 now and he emphasized NOW." The ambulance with Emergency Medical Technicians arrived as Mike was losing consciousness.

We had several frightening experiences but nothing quite as bad as that incident. *Thank you God for Cancer* was not in my vocabulary at that moment.

Lesson learned. As a caregiver, decisions sometimes must be made that will not be well received by the patient.

§

When I told Mike on that particular night that he was going to the hospital he became very agitated and did not want to go. It was an exceptionally cold January night, and I'm sure the idea of getting out of a warm bed wasn't in his plan for the evening.

He was also very weak and had trouble just getting up out of bed for any reason. I am so thankful we went because Mike had become extremely dehydrated and malnourished.

He was given several pints of whole blood, platelets, and many units of fluids. I guess he really needed to go to the hospital. Would he have gone if I had not insisted? –suffice it to say, probably not.

After stabilizing, he was released from the hospital. We came home for exactly three days before he had to return to the hospital. Going back so soon was hard for both of us, and I really began to have a melt down while we were waiting in the emergency room to be admitted.

I made the first of many trips to the Baptist Hospital Chapel. Some of the chaplains came and prayed with me and allowed me to express my feelings, complete with tears.

I am so glad hospitals offer this service. It helped that Mike and I personally knew a few of the men on the pastoral staff. God restored us once again and we continued the dark journey.

§

Journal Entry. His heart rate is still too low, and I get so stressed when the monitor starts beeping. God please help me to be brave.

Scripture for today: *Mark 11:24. Therefore I tell you whatever you ask for in prayer believe that you have received it, and it will be yours*

§

As things progressed and we rode the rollercoaster of highs and lows, I was able to periodically whisper, "Thank you God for cancer and the many lessons learned through this trying time."

My husband has always been a very strong man. He is strong spiritually, mentally and physically. As the chemotherapy treatments continued to build one on the other, they also took their toll on him.

To me, he was turning into someone I didn't even recognize. He lost weight, most of his teeth, and all of his hair. He was always cold because of the blood loss, blood thinners, and just being so weak and thin. He bruised easily and bled a long time with any small wound.

One morning after I got up, I looked into the mirror and didn't recognize myself. Then I looked at him and thought *"Who is that little shriveled man sitting in the living room."*

I began to get worried about myself and my own personal well-being. Depression visited in waves and I don't think it ever totally departed, it just waned a bit. As I had a few minutes of quiet time that same morning, I asked God to help me to continue on this journey. All I had that kept me going had been expended.

Many friends prayed with and for me, and eventually, I cycled out of the feelings of unreality. It was like nothing I have ever felt before and it was very unnerving.

I shared with Mike the things that I was experiencing and as sick as he was he still managed to listen while I talked, cried and just let it all out. I received a lot of encouragement from our talks and managed to keep on going.

One night, Mike and I prayed and begged God to give us a little relief and peace amid the trouble and heartache. God's peace that really does pass our understanding filled our living room and we felt total release. It was a spiritual mountaintop experience for both of us.

§

I am no stranger to the world of cancer. I have been there twice. The first was when I had just turned forty and began having difficulties. My doctor thought it was beginning menopause, but fortunately after telling her some of what was going on she ran tests. I learned that a few cancer cells showed up so a complete hysterectomy was what was needed.

After surgery no further treatment was necessary. I felt very blessed to not have to do chemo or radiation. Among my biggest issues after the surgery was going into a depression.

I was professionally treated and did well for ten years. Once again at my gynecologist's office for a routine exam, I learned the tests showed something suspicious. This time it was colon cancer and was advanced to the point of needing resection surgery and six months of chemo.

It was difficult for me, but I was able to continue working through the time of treatment. A few times I had to call the office and let them know I would be late because of nausea and fatigue. Overall it wasn't a horrible experience for me.

Mike was my caregiver and did a wonderful job of meeting my needs. We never know what might be just around the bend in this life. I'm sure he couldn't imagine ever seeing the tables turned. I honestly was very surprised when we learned he had cancer. Both of his parents lived to be elderly and died of heart related issues.

§

I would like to talk a little about depression at this point. *Depression* for me is a state of low mood and usually manifests itself in an aversion to activity that affects my thoughts, behavior, feelings and sense of well-being.

I and other depressed people can feel sad, anxious, empty, hopeless, helpless, worthless, guilty, irritable or restless. We may lose interest in activities that were once pleasurable, experience loss of appetite or even overeating especially of comfort foods, have problems concentrating, remembering details or making decisions, and may think about, contemplate, attempt or commit suicide. Although I never attempted suicide, I did often think that being dead was better than being alive and in the condition that plagued me.

Insomnia, excessive sleeping, fatigue, aches, pains, digestive problems or reduced energy may also be present. Oftentimes, depression can follow cancer diagnosis and or treatment.

Depression is very difficult to define because it takes on so many forms and is triggered by so many different things. Oftentimes, when in significant depression, colors and illumination becomes intensified, sounds are often irritants, odors are obnoxious, and tasks are insurmountable.

It bothers me when I hear well-meaning people, especially preachers, say that depression is always spiritual and practicing a ritual of Scriptural memorization and quotation will send it away. That just is not true, and I am sure that those words can easily roll off the tongues of those who have never suffered clinical depression versus spiritual depression.

When I had surgery and was placed on steroids, I went into a deep depression, rolled up in the fetal position, stayed there and cried. Only the care of a psychiatrist and antidepressants brought me out of it, after I stopped taking the steroids.

Depression has occasionally robbed me of the joy of my salvation and caused me to doubt my relationship with Jesus. There were times when I didn't feel loved, accepted, or saved.

Working through and with depression is a challenge that I pray you will never have to experience. I often felt like throwing in the towel and running away. Those were the times when I had to rely on that promise that *I could do anything through Christ Who strengthened me.* There were times when He would literally carry me through a task, hold me up, move my hands, and think for me.

Frustration and depression go hand in hand. Frustration can often be overcome by success in a task. Depression on the other hand isn't impressed by success and has no sympathy for failure.

I am happy to report that at this point I am depression free with only short visits from my old friend.

§

Before ending this chapter, I want to describe for you how bad our situation was just before the Lord stepped in and worked some miracles in both our lives.

Mike was facing major surgery and possibly a craniotomy to remove tumor tissue from his sinus area. I had developed an unusual colon issue where uncontrollable diarrhea for days stopped my activities and trips to the doctor's office did not help. I lost ten pounds, became weak, and was rendered nearly immobile, and we could not even attend church.

On one rare occasion when the diarrhea stopped, we attended a Sunday evening service at Bellevue Baptist Church. They offer a James Ministry after the evening service where anyone who requests it can be anointed with oil and be prayed for by the ministerial staff for a healing. Both Mike and I were anointed that night and the staff laid hands on us and prayed for us.

The next day, a friend took me to lunch and while at lunch I became ill. There is an old hymn by William Cowper that says *God moves in a mysterious way, His wonders to perform...*

My friend took me home and told me on the way that she had suffered the exact same symptoms and that her doctor had prescribed a certain medication that healed her of the issue.

I immediately called my Gastro Intestinal doctor who prescribed the meds, and in two days, the ordeal was over.

Mike will tell of his surgery, and we will both testify to the power of having been anointed with oil and prayed for.

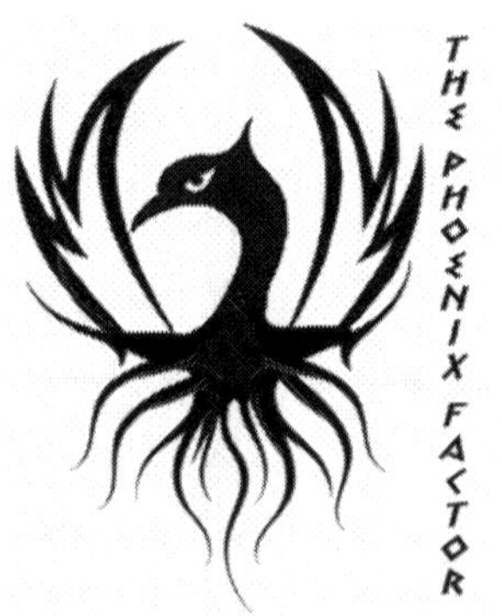

I can say beyond the shadow of a doubt that I am thankful that we were able to make it through this ordeal. We did survive and we are better people for the journey.

My ability to handle very difficult and often repulsive tasks has been enhanced and I have learned to rise to whatever the occasion requires of me.

§§§

Chapter Three

The Good, the Bad, the Ugly

> *Psalm 30:5. 5b Weeping may stay for the night, but rejoicing comes in the morning.*

And we will weep, especially in the darkness of the night, but we can hope for the joy of the morning that will come with the sunrise.

§

Mike. As we opened this book, we laid out for you an overview of many of the harsh, frightening, and uncomfortable things that happen to a cancer survivor as he or she fights for survival.

Now we want to provide things we feel will be of help in your personal journey on that path that might prove to be not so dark because you had a guide that has gone before you.

Although brutal, graphic, and sometimes almost surreal, what we will address now you need to know, can take strength from, and find encouragement in the fact that others have made it through and have come out on the other side.

§

Please allow me to begin by saying that we should listen to and pay attention to our bodies as they try to tell us that something is amiss, and we should seek the services and counsel of experts.

There's an old adage that goes, "The doctor who treats himself has a fool for a patient". That is also true of the patient who treats or diagnoses himself. Remember the words of that wise little elf, Puck.

We all should be well-versed in a variety of subjects, including health care. But this can lead to denial, misidentification, and ultimately, it can allow a serious ailment to gain strength past the point of early intervention.

I had trouble swallowing for two years along with increasing sinus trouble. I took my complaint to four doctors over a six month period. None of them could see anything wrong. I finally went to see my family physician who was on vacation, but whose nurse practitioner examined me, and within five minutes, was setting me up with an ear, nose, and throat specialist.

§

Before we go any further, we need to consider the emotions that may come to play immediately with the delivery of a cancer diagnosis as well as throughout the course of treatment. They increase with the passing of time as you have the opportunity to evaluate and think.

The following table is not meant to be all inclusive, but after interviewing over a hundred cancer patients and families, it provides a pretty good idea what you may be facing. Just know that others have experienced these things.

Because of the several different dominant personality types, individuals usually find themselves with different emotions or sets of feelings that are stronger in some people than in others.

Anger	Disappointment	Guilt	Panic
Anguish	Disgust	Helplessness	Rage
Anxiety	Dismay	Hopelessness	Rejection
Apathy	Distrust	Hurt	Sadness
Bitterness	Dread	Indignation	Self Pity
Confusion	Emptiness	Isolation	Shock
Denial	Envy	Lethargy	Stress
Depression	Fear	Loneliness	Uncertainty
Despair	Grief	Lovelessness	Worthlessness

We don't want to sound preachy in this or any other area, but there is a baseline that we should strive to achieve as we ride the emotional rollercoaster that cancer brings into our lives.

As believers, we all deal with negative emotions that do affect our spiritual well-being and physical health and healing in a bad way. It will help early on to deal with them according to Scripture and the encouragement of those who have gone before.

In Galatians 5, the apostle Paul tells us that all believers have and can exhibit what is called *the fruit of the Holy Spirit* who resides within them.

These include *love, joy, patience, peace, kindness, goodness, gentleness, faithfulness and self-control.* All of these things will come to play at sometime in your journey.

In *Romans 12,* he mentions that we are not to be conformed to the values of the secular world but be transformed by the renewing of our minds through Scripture. This is how we can deal with our emotions more effectively.

Alcohol, recreational drugs, and prescription medication when abused will not bring lasting relief (they might kill you when mixed with cancer treatment protocols), but they will negatively impact one's overall well-being.

In other words, what might knock the socks off a human being who is not a believer, can be better managed with God's help. Maybe not in a fun way, but in a way that will allow us to make it through and exit the dark tunnel into the sunshine at the end.

A negative attitude slows and impedes healing as well as accelerates the harmful effects of cancer. This really reminds me of a term not too much in vogue today, but is really appropriate to attitude and how it impacts healing.

Psychosomatic. Right out of the dictionary is defined as: *something mentally induced and describes a physical illness that is caused by mental factors such as stress or the effects related to such illnesses.*

This area relates to the mind and body. It involves both the mind and body, and I must add also the spirit.

For example, anger is among the most devastating emotions. It ranges from mild irritation or frustration to outright rage or fury. It precipitates violence and irreparably harms relationships.

Some patients direct their anger at their family, the doctors and medical staff, or at God. Family, even spouses may be angry with the patient for getting sick and disrupting their lives. And believe me folks, cancer does disrupt lives.

Anger is a very normal reaction to the stress a family feels during diagnosis and treatment. It is important to find an outlet, such as talking to someone, meditating, playing a favorite game, etc., in order to relieve the potentially destructive tension. Judy and I have played hundreds of games of electronic scrabble.

Both patients and their families including support persons need support and escape from the drudgery of all that cancer and treatment bring to the table.

We included the subject of anger because like all emotions it can be appropriately handled with the excellent books and helps that abound on-line and at booksellers. The one thing that I can't overemphasize here is clinging to hope.

Simply put, hope is the belief that a positive outcome lies ahead of your trial and challenges. Hope is also being honest with yourself about your situation, while looking forward to positive outcomes in your future. If you loose sight of hope, you will pay a heavy price in your overall mental and physical well-being.

§

Cancer has been a challenging but interesting journey into the depths of darkness, suffering, faith, our relationship with God and each other. Please allow me to introduce the somewhat extraordinary beginning of my personal story.

I have been a Christian, Bible and Sunday School teacher, deacon, personal witness, and lay minister for about forty-five years, mostly with the help of my precious wife, Judy.

A little over a year ago, I found myself at a place in my personal walk with Jesus where I was dissatisfied with the depth and breadth of our relationship and asked Him to take me deeper and allow me to feel His presence and love in ways I have never before experienced them.

I promised the Lord that I would do whatever He asked, and go wherever He led me. This all came just before a sermon by our pastor in which he encouraged the congregation to *trust Jesus, no matter what.*

On a side note, someone once said, “Be careful what you ask for, you might just get it.” This became fleshed out in a way I will never forget.

Now let me explain at this point that I do not believe that Jesus gave me cancer; this corrupt, disease filled, cursed world gave me the disease. He already knew my condition; I had developed cancer –trust Jesus.

My Lord told me in no uncertain terms that I was going to experience cancer and suffer a lot, but that I would not die. He also let me know that I would bring Him glory, reflect His love to others, and be an encouragement to those with whom I previously had no real empathy.

When the Lord of Glory and omnipotent King tells you that you are going to suffer, you should listen to Him.

When I could no longer breathe through my nose or swallow, I found myself in the office of my Ear, Nose and Throat doctor. A few days later, I was having tests, MRI’s, CT Scans, and all the rest.

Here is where I began to realize just how much control that Jesus had over this whole process. I am, or was seriously claustrophobic.

The disorder manifested itself in the past during MRI’s, especially the older type units where I would be stuffed into a tube that touched my arms and sides and prompted my memory of Edgar Allen Poe's works, such as Premature Burial.

Now, here I was again, only this time I had the added stress of knowing I probably had cancer. No amount of Scripture had helped me get through the MRIs of the past. I cried, prayed, tried visualization, and everything else I could think of to no avail.

This time, as I lay on my back and had the retainer mask placed over my head, as I have said earlier, I began praying. Praying to Jesus, to my Lord, to my King, just didn't seem to fit the situation.

Then I remembered the words of *Romans 8:15. The Spirit you received does not make you slaves, so that you live in fear again; rather, the Spirit you received brought about your adoption to sonship. And by him we cry, "Abba, Father."*

That's when I began to weep and cry out in my mind, *Abba, Father, Daddy, I can't take this, your child is losing it, please help me.*

The human mind is a marvelous yet strange and often unfathomable thing. I knew I had about forty-five minutes to be in that infernal machine.

Then, it was as though I left my circumstances. I looked up and coming down from the ceiling was Jesus. Yes, He looked like the pictures I had seen of artists' conceptions with the red sash around his white robe, holding his right hand up as he descended to me.

I raised my right hand up to Him and he took my hand. I don't know how I raised my right hand even though I was in the MRI tube. But I felt myself rise from the tube and the next thing I knew, Jesus and I were walking in what I think was the Garden of Eden in all its beauty and wonders.

We talked as we walked, but I don't remember the subjects we discussed. Then, in a moment, in the twinkling of an eye, the slab was being rolled out of the tube and I was finished, and Jesus was gone, and I missed Him.

I doubted my own experience until I later spoke with a friend of long standing, and he told me he had a similar experience when he was strapped into a rotating bed after heart surgery where he stayed for two months.

Charlie Biggs may be my biggest supporter and encourager. He is a wonderful Christian man whom I believe only the prayers of a lot of people kept him from dying during and after five bypasses with numerous complications.

One more thing before I leave this remarkable event. I had another MRI two months later without a twinge of claustrophobia. Pretty neat I'd say –trust Jesus.

This is only one of several spiritual miracle-like experiences I encountered in my dark journey. We'll talk about the others as we move on.

A few days after the results came back, and through the use of a special camera and scope, I saw the tumors. I then found myself in the hospital where the fun really began –trust Jesus.

§

As my Otolaryngology; Head and Neck Surgeon put it, "We can't chance doing a biopsy on the tumor at the base of the tongue because it may swell, cutting off your breathing. We have to perform a temporary tracheotomy and insert a breathing tube to provide a secondary breathing path. We will remove it when it has fulfilled its purpose." By the way, that would be seven months later.

What the doctor told me just before surgery introduced me to the world of modern medicine and its sometimes brutal yet necessary processes.

He could not put me to sleep under general anesthesia for the surgery, because the muscles that keep my throat open might relax, cutting off my breathing due to the size of the tumor.

So, it would be done with a local anesthetic, permitting me to watch and experience the whole procedure –trust Jesus.

The local anesthesia worked pretty well, but it felt like a giant wasp was stinging my throat as it was injected. It did allow me to watch as the surgery was performed and a large hole was cut into my throat and then cauterized sending smoke signals of my burning flesh into the air.

As seven or eight student physicians looked on, I apprehensively allowed the procedure to progress until finally the trach was inserted and blessed general anesthesia was administered allowing me to sleep through the biopsy of my sinus cavity and tongue.

Waking up with a trach sticking out of my throat was somewhat of a nightmare. I started coughing up bloody slime as soon as I awoke sufficiently to know what was going on.

Now we are not talking about a little slime here and there. We are talking about the ugly ooze being shot out of the trach under pressure all over the place.

The bloody slime would remain an issue for the entire time I hosted the trach, but it did subside to manageable amounts as the weeks passed and my body accepted the foreign matter in my throat.

My mind also had to accept the device, and that came with time, experience, and learning to function with it. It became quite uncomfortable at times and a cough impulse was always present when we serviced the unit.

Cleaning and maintaining the trach would become a significant and disgusting task that was performed by my care-giving wife despite the unpleasant steps in the once-a-day ritual.

Many things would be done by Judy for which she had no previous experience. In cancer care giving, one has to be prepared for just about anything.

Learning to live with, speak, vomit, adjust, replace the gauze buffer between the unit and my neck, and use of the Passy-Muir® Valve through which I spoke without having to cover the trach tube with a finger, would remain significant challenges.

The discomforts, dangers, requirements, and irritations surrounding the use of a trach all acted as constant reminders to pray for the day it would be removed. Once inserted, however, the doctor will make absolutely sure that removing it is the right thing to do.

The tracheostomy or tracheotomy stands as a monument to the beginning of our headlong dive into cancer for my first time. When the biopsies returned, they bore out the fact that I indeed had Squamous cell carcinoma.

The rest of the story will reveal numerous lessons learned, life truths, and the tenuousness life itself and the things we hold as precious and necessary to our personal comfort. One thing that I feel is significant at this juncture is that we can all practice patience and consideration of others, even though we are not on top of our game, so to speak.

As I close this chapter, it is with many reflections of the good, the bad, and the ugly in what I have come to call my Grand Prix start in the race for a cure to my cancer. I must say in retrospect, we are not alone in the fight.

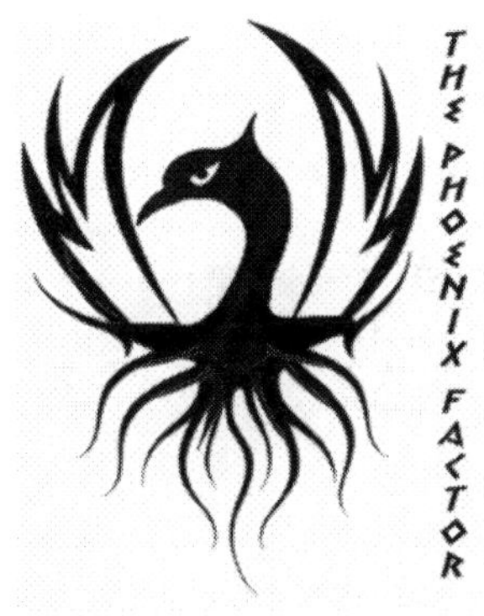

We humans expend a great deal of effort and resources trying to ensure our comfort, pleasure, and access to the many luxuries at our disposal.

I have found that modern medicine, and the most caring and competent doctors, care less about our comfort and more about saving or enhancing our physical lives.

For those who are caught up in privacy and all it has to offer, health care often comes at the expense of comfort, dignity, and modesty.

As a cancer survivor, I and my myriad brothers and sisters in the family of abnormal cell disorders, have yielded many rights to comfort and luxury in our quest to stay alive and to have a fighting chance to beat what may be the world's most prevalent disease.

We all must come to grips, and have patience with discomfort, pain, nausea, medical devices, scheduling nightmares, and medication and treatment side effects.

Patience and a positive attitude will enhance our chances of survival. In the long run, the traits we develop throughout our journey will enhance life in general.

§

Scripture Verse. Isaiah 41:10, *So do not fear, for I am with you; do not be dismayed, for I am your God. I will strengthen you and help you; I will uphold you with my righteous right hand.*

§§§

Chapter Four

Which Way is Up

James 1:12. Blessed is the one who perseveres under trial because, having stood the test, that person will receive the crown of life that the Lord has promised to those who love him.

There will be times when you will not know who you are or which way is up. You will ask yourself, "Will this ever end?"

Perseverance is a trait that must be grown and nurtured, but will produce patience through trials and suffering and will provide the key to finishing your personal race.

§

As I journeyed deeper into the great and dark chasm of confusion, distress, frustration, and lost more and more control of my life, I forgot who I had been and then didn't know who I was.

Cancer diagnosis, treatment, and follow-up can be a lot like the old Chinese water torture that we have all heard about. It is a process in which water is slowly dripped onto a person's forehead, allegedly driving the restrained victim insane. This form of torture has been around and documented as early as the 15th century.

One small irritation or disappointment after another in rapid succession, seemingly unending, until the patient loses it or as they say today, *freaks out*. It happened to me, and I don't know too many patients that have not experienced this to some degree.

Very few people are equipped to handle a cancer diagnosis, and even fewer for a prognosis of how many months remain in one's life due to an aggressive and terminal type of cancer.

So what is the answer? It's possible to make it through cancer, chemotherapy, radiation, surgery, medication, radiofrequency ablation, and the side effects of all of them.

This table can help draw into focus the answers from the One who called Himself "I Am." Compared with who I saw myself to be; God revealed himself as who He is.

You will not, hopefully, experience all of these, but it is possible that you might. Be prepared, be willing to fight, be open to help and encouragement, keep an open mind, pray, and capitalize on your personal relationship with Jesus.

There will come to play several factors in the way one feels and responds to the emotional train wreck that can and often does occur in the soul of a cancer patient and survivor.

Chemical or medicine reactions or side effects, abnormal highs and lows, starvation induced euphoria or lethargy, overdoses of prescribed medications for sleep, blood thinners, anti-depressants, etc., can all be contributors to our feelings.

If we add these to the actual psychological implications of cancer treatment, it is understandable how the items in this table could come to be.

I feel	**God is**	**Comment**
Unloved and unwanted	Love *1 John 4:8*	Unconditional love does not exist without God
Great turmoil	Peace *John 14:27*	God gives what pills cannot
Incapable	Grace *Romans 1:7*	God is never overextended
Sad and downtrodden	Joy *Romans 15:13*	Joy is forever, happiness fades
Weak	Strength *Psalm 28:7*	Can't walk? God will carry you
Grave danger	Safety *Psalm 91:1-4*	You can't buy better armor
Lost	Shelter *Psalm 46:1-2*	God is the ultimate storm shelter
Overwhelmed	Creator *Genesis 1:1*	He made and understands it all
Distraught	Comforter *2 Corinthians 1:6*	Let it all hang out with God
This is never ending	The Beginning and the End *Revelation 22:13*	God knew you had cancer before you did, and He knows the ending
Incompetent	The Way, the Truth, the Light *John 14:6*	You needn't stumble in the dark
Hungry but cannot eat	The Bread of Life *John 6:35*	The body, soul, and spirit all hunger
Healing is not for me	The Healer *Exodus 15:26*	Doctors practice medicine; healing comes from God

§

So here I am, lying in a hospital bed, shooting bloody ooze from my trach, IVs infusing life sustaining fluids into my body, preventing dehydration that could kill me, not knowing what to expect.

Since I was a patient in a teaching institution, I didn't know it at the time, but I would see nineteen doctors and their entourages of students, coming and going at all hours, for the entire time I was there. That turned out to be over three weeks –trust Jesus.

Bless her heart, my beloved was there with me the whole time, and I know she felt helpless as she watched her husband succumb to the scientific but mostly heartless protocols of a cancer treatment ward in a university hospital.

General surgeons, radiation specialists, oncologists, ENTs, oral surgeons, pulmonologists, hepatologists, hematologists, radiologists, endocrinologists, wound specialists, dieticians, nephrologists, physical therapists, respiratory therapists, nurses (thank you Jesus for nurses), anesthesia doctors, operating room staffs, X-ray, CT, MRI, and ultra-sound technicians, patient transporters of varying degrees of skill, and the precious people who cleaned my room, body, and took care of habitability items, all jockeyed for our time.

Needless to say, we lost scope of who was in charge, because each new doctor said that he or she was. That is not meant to be a joke, and it wasn't funny.

I am going to summarize what happened next in a way that will help you understand how absolute despair can creep into this already nerve wracking scenario.

In the next twelve hours, we would be counseled, subjected to, informed and directed by, educated and programmed by the doctors who would invade, deform, modify, and subject my body to things done in the name of science and medicine that would fit easily into the old science fiction horror movies where Doctor Frankenstein builds his monster.

And we were supposed to agree and accept the following with complete confidence in what the doctors ordered.

Before I could return home, the treatment team would pull all my teeth to prepare for radiation because that procedure would make my jaw bones brittle and they might break if I had to have a tooth pulled.

Next, I would be prepped for radiation by having a mud mask poured over my face while I held a breathing tube in my mouth, allowing it to set up.

The mask would then be adapted to radiation points and would be bolted over my head for each treatment to hold me still until the radiation could be targeted and completed. This would be repeated twenty, forty, sixty, or hundreds of times, or however many treatments it might take.

I would be prepped for surgery on my tongue and sinus cavities which would be tantamount to removing a large portion of my tongue, cutting into and peeling my nose back to allow entrance into the sinus cavity to scrape out the tumor tissue.

The next big revelation was the chemotherapy treatment that would comprise three of the strongest chemo chemicals available, one at a time, three in a row until my kidneys and liver began to shut down, at which time they would stop the treatment until my creatinine levels, that measured my kidney functions, returned to a safe level.

That was not the end of the stressors introduced into my already weakening constitution. Now we will look at what I could expect as side effects from it all.

The expert physicians that specialize in all the aspects of the prescribed treatment protocols briefed Judy and me about what we could expect from chemotherapy, radiation, and surgery.

From the chemotherapy, I could expect some or all of the following side effects.

- Loss of hair from all over my body
- Loss of taste
- Food revulsion
- Nausea
- Weakness
- Dizziness
- Lethargy
- Kidney and liver function reduction
- Weight loss
- Muscle loss
- Blood clots
- Being cold with chills
- Passing out
- Dehydration
- Mouth fungus and blisters called thrush or oropharyngeal candidiasis, or OPC, a yeast infection that develops in the mouth, throat, and on the tongue
- Immune system weakening
- Diarrhea
- Constipation
- Frequent urination
- Etc.

From the radiation, we could expect

- Hearing and vision loss
- Loss of taste
- Inability to swallow
    - With this there is a very real probability of aspiration pneumonia or bronchopneumonia that develops due to the entrance of foreign materials into the bronchial tree, usually oral or gastric contents including food, saliva, or nasal secretions.
- Need for a feeding tube
- Burning soreness in the throat
- Cancer
- Long-term toxicity
- Radioactivity
- Never sing again because my voice box would be fried
- Gravel voice
- Etc.

Surgery has its own side effects that would be in addition to those already mentioned.

- Removal of tongue mass
- Scarring
- Loss of smell
- Brain leakage of spinal fluids
- Seizures
- Anti seizure medication long term
- Staph infection, et al
- Extended healing time
- Etc.

§

As we returned to our room, we had been officially programmed into all the above protocols without even being asked if we agreed or wanted to opt out of all or any of them.

That night Judy and I crashed big time as our minds and spirits went into overload, and our lives as we knew them just vaporized into an unknown future filled with frightening possibilities.

§

The next thing I knew, I was signing surgery documents and was on my way to oral surgery to have my teeth extracted –all my teeth.

I had the presence of mind to stop the world at that time. I had already had surgery for the biopsies, tracheostomy, and the placement of a peripherally inserted central catheter or PICC or PIC line, a form of intravenous access used for a prolonged chemotherapy regimen. I said I would keep my top six and bottom six front teeth and just risk it.

§

After the surgery, I experienced a problem, and for thirty minutes complained to the recovery room nurse that I couldn't breathe. This prompted a pulmonary team to come to the recovery room and scope my lungs, from which they discovered an occlusion –trust Jesus.

An occlusion of the upper lungs is the closing, obstructing or bringing together of a passageway. When the upper lungs are occluded, air, or in some cases, blood vessels, cannot pass through as is necessary for lung function.

There are various types of occlusions that may occur in the lungs and the consequences that can result range in severity from mild discomfort to death. I did get to experience an occlusion being removed from my lung while I was awake.

I then found myself back in my room with my mouth full of stitches and more stressed than before.

§

The mind is a remarkable synergy of experiential knowledge and related emotions. It is housed in the brain and central nervous system, and will follow us to heaven when we die, so it must also reside in the soul and spirit –maybe.

It does, however have a breaking point where it snaps and can no longer normally process experiences. That is what happened to Judy and me on that night, in our room.

About three o'clock in the morning, I was already awake. I sat up and placed my head on the rolling serving tray by my bed. It was a surreal moment as I was no longer in control of anything remotely connected with being in charge of my life –as though we ever really are.

Images began to dart in an out of my mind like so many specters of things past and future. I felt like my life was over and that I had no future.

Here is the kicker, as they say. I associated my worth by who I had been, what I looked like, my mental acuity, and my capacity to make money and care for my family.

What I saw of myself for the future was a sickly old man, bone skinny, hairless, wobbling like a Weeble as I tried to walk, never eating again, throwing up all the time, and unable to ever be happy or joyful. Then the dam broke.

I again cried out to my Abba, Father, Daddy, and I begged Him to help me make it through this ordeal. I was shaking and hopeless when it happened.

I was born prematurely at seven months and was a sickly baby and toddler. I threw up a lot and was just a puny kid. Do you know what came to my mind? Of course you don't, you haven't read that part yet.

As I hugged the commode and vomited violently, my mother would come into the bathroom and place a cool wet wash cloth over the back of my neck. Her presence and that wash cloth did not make me well, but it calmed me with an assurance that this was not going to last forever. As a three or four year-old toddler, I remember that.

§

As I prayed, the room became even quieter than it had been and the darkness was dispelled by a sort of illuminated mist. It was as though my mother's hand was on the back of my neck and peace fell on me. It was the kind of peace that surpasses all understanding.

Something changed in me. The challenges were still there, but my head was clear and I felt like there was light at the end of the tunnel for me.

I felt my Lord's presence in that room, I sensed his encouragement. My faith in Him turned into a kind of sight and sensing that filled the room.

The message that I received in my mind and heart was that no matter what I went through, what I would become on the other side, what my limitations might be, my Lord was with me and would use me for His glory. He also said, "Trust Me." There was that phrase again –trust Jesus.

Then it was over and morning light had broken, and I felt empowered to take the next step. I actually began thinking clear thoughts about researching, being selective, and being in charge of what would happen to me. The bottom line was that my pity party was over –at least for now.

§

As that morning progressed, we received two visitors; two long-time friends, church family actually. Doctor Stan and Carol Crunk were on their way from his sister's home. She had just died of Sarcoma cancer, yet, here they were visiting me, and they had brought a gift.

Stan had personally received a book entitled "When God & Cancer Meet" by Lynn Eib. He said that he couldn't wait to bring it to me because it had meant so much to him while battling his own cancer. Stan had renal cell carcinoma and malignant melanoma.

His treatment was surgery and radiofrequency ablation. That is a medical term for burning out the cancer with electricity. On another note, Stan's remaining sister has been diagnosed with pancreatic cancer. Stan and his wife, Carole are an expert cancer survivor and care giver team.

After an encouraging visit, we prayed together, they departed, and I was left with the book that would change the way I looked at my own situation.

I tried reading Lynn's book, but could not get through the first chapter. I was still dealing with the reality and acceptance of what was happening to me.

It would be weeks before I could read it. But when Judy and I read it together aloud at home, our thoughts changed as did our reality.

One of the strengths of When God & Cancer Meet is the fact that Lynn Eib is a cancer survivor and writes from experience, not just from interviews and hearsay.

That formed an immediate bond between her and her readers. We'll speak more of Lynn's excellent work as we progress in this book.

Thousands of people were praying for Judy and me. Entire churches of differing denominations, friends, family, even an Episcopal convent were praying. I'll share a bit later how prayer changed things for us.

One of our dearest long-time friends, Sheila Harrell brought gifts and goodies several times, but one thing she did for us was to help Judy set up a social media page designed to share our situation with friends, acquaintances, and interested parties.

That tool proved to be priceless and actually gave Judy a lot of control over communicating prayer needs, updates, setbacks, and progress. Thanks Sheila, you are an angel.

We need to include a word on the importance of friends. We had close friends that stood by us during the entire process and maintained contact with us through it all. A few very special people come to mind above all the rest.

Our best friends Jimmy and Renate Wood, Faye Russell, Sheila Harrell, Charlie Biggs, Vicky Evans, Walter and Martha Edwards, and our Branson friends Ray and Sonia Tucker and Paul, Annette and Nicole Yendez who kept things together for us at our home in Kimberling City all deserve honorable mention and our sincere gratitude for being there.

Good and faithful friends don't wear out over the long run. They hang in there when the going gets really tough. And each of the above did just that.

§

There was a period for me when I had been told I had cancer, I relinquished control of my life and aspirations, resigned myself to my circumstances, and accepted the fact that everything was about to, or has already begun to change.

The hardest part of all this was knowing that things would probably never be the same again. To me that was a bad thing; I have subsequently learned that it is not necessarily a bad thing.

The worst part of it all is when we become rigid and refuse to change, accept the inevitable, and try our best to stand defiantly against the hurricane force winds of life altering trials.

That is when we find that even the strongest and largest oak tree sometimes snaps and falls because it refuses to bend like the smaller but more flexible pine tree.

§

There is an old hymn that says, *"It is no secret, what God can do. What He's done for others, He'll do for you."* It is the veterans of the battle with cancer that can best tell us all what God can do.

§

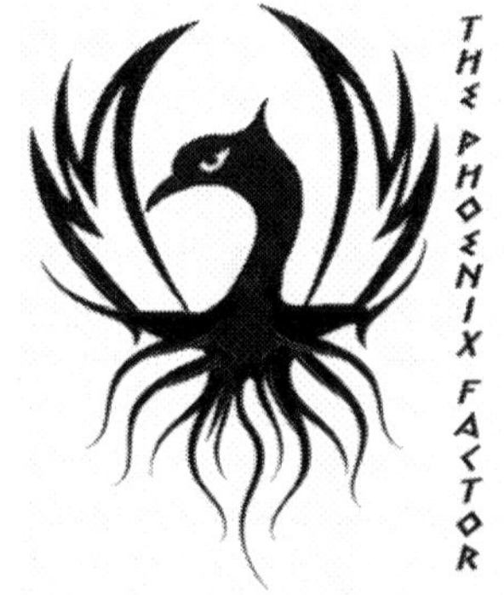

Cancer survivors have all experienced similar disappointments, challenges, fears, struggles, and frustrations.

They are the best sources of encouragement, hope, education, recommendations, and hope for the future. They are treasures to hold near and dear in the journey toward restored health.

§

Scripture Verse. *Jeremiah 29: 1-13.* [11]*For I know the plans*
I have for you," declares the LORD*, "plans to prosper you*
and not to harm you, plans to give you hope and a future.
[12]*Then you will call on me and come and pray to me, and I*
will listen to you. [13]*You will seek me and find me when you*
seek me with all your heart.

§§§

Chapter Five

It Just Keeps Getting Better

Each of my attending specialists, of course, had his or her unique personality and bedside manner. I liked and felt confident with them all except for one doctor.

All the while the newly assigned specialist spoke to me; it became apparent that the doctor was missing one main thing –a heart. The information was cold, clinical, and failed to establish any kind of bond of trust or credibility.

We were dictated to about what protocols would be employed and what we could expect. The more the doctor spoke, the more my heart sank until finally I stopped the conversation. I addressed the doctor with direct eye contact, in a firm monotone approach.

"Doctor, do you realize that you are talking to a human being and not a lab rat?" Do you realize I have feelings, fears, apprehensions, and need some reassurance, especially from you."

The good doctor wasn't ready for that and put forth a half hearted apology before leaving somewhat flustered.

§

Going home was a moving target for us. Each time we were given a departure date, it changed –four times in three weeks. Finally, I opted out of radiation. You might ask why?

We do not intend to try to dissuade anyone from following the doctor's recommendations, but I do say you need to call the shots as much as possible. We used our laptop devices and the hospital broadband hot spot to research radiation.

Our friends communicated information about their loved ones and acquaintances, everyone prayed fervently for us. Considering all the facts and their input, we made a decision on what we determined would be in our best interests.

So we opted to begin the chemotherapy regimen the next day –that proved challenging. The treatment consisted of massive doses of three different chemo's every day, all day until the third day when my kidneys and liver began to fail –trust Jesus.

The treatment was stopped and the specialists began monitoring me to make sure I didn't die. I did take a significant interest in test results for the first time in my life.

Violent diarrhea, nausea, dizziness, weakness, and extreme yuck, all became my closest friends. Four days after the treatment stopped, I forced myself into the shower to clean my body, and all my hair fell out except a few defiant stragglers. What a mess that proved to be, especially when I tried to rinse off my former very thick mop of hair.

The nurses (again, thank you Jesus, for nurses) administered blood thinners, fluids, then platelets, and then got seriously on my case when they found me shaving with a safety razor. I guess if I had cut myself, I would have bled big time.

After three weeks of hospitalization, we went home with a list of to do's as long as my arm. We were transferred to West Cancer Clinic for treatment, monitoring, scans, and supervision by a new oncologist –our first very bright spot in a long time.

§

As a new patient, standing outside a very modern, brightly painted, well kept building waiting to enter West Cancer Clinic, I looked around at the people that were coming and going in wheelchairs, walkers, being assisted by family members, and those who walked slowly, but on their own without support devices.

I found out later that this two-story building comprised 52,359 square feet of inside space; was surrounded on three sides by 272 parking spaces; and hosted 225 employees. But those statistics were not what made this building and grounds special. It was the spirit, professionalism, kindness, mercy, and heart that were manifested by the medical, technical, administrative, and volunteer staff that makes up West Cancer Clinic.

I would progressively learn that this scientific yet sacred place was a bastion of defense against an enemy so aggressive and large that, if left unchecked, could wipe out the human race by itself over a few generations.

My primary oncologist is with the West Cancer Treatment Clinic in Memphis, Tennessee. He is a gentle soul with genuine feelings and a considerate spirit that allows him to see his patients as real people.

He was recommended to us by our Primary Care Physician. He cared for our family doctor's mother until her death from cancer shortly before we met him. We are both thankful that he was placed in our path as we journeyed on into the throes of cancer's overwhelming hold.

He explained that the treatment he was prescribing would be brutal and I would be very sick and uncomfortable during the process. Since each patient is different, it is impossible to tell just how anyone will respond to the treatment. Suffice it to say that chemotherapy is not an exact science but is more educated touch and go.

He was right. It was his firm but gentle coaching that directed us through the next nine months of treatment and subsequent follow ups.

§

I need to inject something here that is important and you will experience it to some degree. It isn't rejection; you are not a leper needing a cow bell around your neck and yelling out "unclean" wherever you go. But you might feel that way sometimes.

The first night I was home, my son, daughter-in-law, and two granddaughters came over to see me. I was of course in my recliner, balding head, and trach sticking out of my throat.

My youngest granddaughter, Aria Quinne wouldn't come near me even when I asked her. That just about broke my heart. I had to pull away and think until I realized that people just don't know how to handle a cancer patient.

It pretty much stayed that way until the trach came out seven months later –trust Jesus.

§

Let's stop for a moment and look at some giants among men and women. Let's recognize the real overcomers, who give of themselves to others, who share positive testimonies with whoever will listen, and bare their souls without restraint if the situation merits.

These angels of mercy and love are the aged ones, the young ones, the terminal patients, the frail, weak, and wasting ones who have little left to give, but give anyway.

I have held their hands, hugged their necks, sat and prayed with them, shared chemo stories, and gave them copies of Lynn Eib's book. They call me at home, smile when they see me coming, and share their hearts as though I were family –and I am.

Some of these hall-of-famers become survivors, some succumb to the disease, and some go deeper into the treatment until they are just above flat-lining.

I've said my last goodbyes to some, while others hold on with all that is in them. They have each and every one been blessings to my wife and me.

When the mythological Death Angel comes for them, they usually go willingly with a smile of relief. Oh, they look out and back to what they are leaving behind with sadness and remorse for having to depart, but with happy anticipation of what awaits them on arrival in their new home.

I feel I am on holy ground as I try to minister to these beloveds, and always feel the Lord's presence with me and the ones I am there to serve. There have been very few jerks to which I have ministered on the way.

There are a few bitter ones, but most have had an opportunity to allow cancer and God to tenderize their hearts and soften their spirits.

Judy and I are indebted to the cancer survivors who have gone before us and paved the way for us to come later. There is a glow, almost like an aura or halo around the face of patients on maintenance –who are being kept alive by treatments. Once you begin speaking with them and they start sharing their testimony, you won't want to leave.

I received a great deal of peace and reassurance from these veteran cancer survivors. The wisdom they shared, the recommendations they offered, the advice they were always willing to provide really made a difference in our own struggles.

§

I am really thankful for my *port* or *portacath;* a small medical appliance that is installed beneath the skin. A catheter connects the port to a vein.

Just under the skin, the port has a septum through which drugs can be injected and blood samples may be drawn many times, usually with much less discomfort for me than the more typical needle stick.

Ports are used to treat most oncology patients I have met that have been around awhile. They are usually inserted in the upper chest, into the *superior vena cava,* a large diameter yet short vein that carries deoxygenated blood from the upper half of the body to the heart's right atrium, just below the clavicle or collar bone.

Well, I am one of those poor souls that if it can go wrong, with me it will go wrong. Because of the trach, I was disrobed, prepped, and then released without the surgeon being able to insert the port twice with success on the third attempt.

They found I had a blood clot in my upper or superior vena cava, so on the third try, they used the lower or inferior vena cava and I finally had my own port. However, it was painful and disheartening to go through all that.

It doesn't stop there, however. On the first use of my brand new port, the phlebotomist stuck me five times trying to access the port and insert the Huber needle. When you see a patient with a yellow and clear tubular apparatus sticking out of their shirt or blouse, that's what it is. That's where they will be hooked up for infusion. On the fifth time, I passed out and stayed out for about ten minutes.

I woke up throwing up all over the place, in a bed in the back of the clinic. That won me a trip to the hospital where it was discovered that I was dehydrated and in need of whole blood. Being admitted by my doctor got me into a room very quickly, for which I was grateful.

Allow me to mention that having a port means that a line runs into one's heart through a vein and so it must be treated as a foreign object and there might be some feelings that go along with its presence.

Dehydration is an ever-present condition that can cause serious problems and even death. We learned to seek intervention as I manifested certain signs of impending system crashes. The most insidious harbingers of the condition are lethargy, slow pulse, low blood pressure, and losing consciousness.

We learned that by going to West Clinic daily if necessary, and being infused with fluids can ward off the effects of dehydration.

§

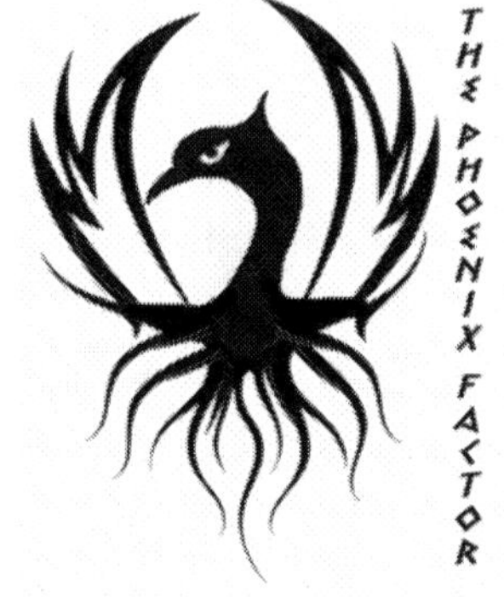

Usually we will not seek out paths that lead through pain, fear, the unknown, or those which lead us out of our comfort zone.

Changes in our regimen require adjustment. Learning to cope with and live through discomfort; practicing love, kindness and mercy while feeling yucky, may not seem desirable, but their outcome is surprisingly positive.

I can testify that those things help us to grow into more tolerant and resilient people. *Besides, when we stop hurting and become less nauseous, it feels so good!*

§§§

Chapter Six

An Oasis in a Desert of Desperation

A strange phenomenon develops with many patients of West Cancer Treatment Center, and I am sure other centers as well. Even though West Clinic is the place where so many people get so sick from the treatments, it becomes a type of Mecca for the patients.

After a while, we feel like we need a fix. We need the fellowship of others like us. We thrive on the free coffee, snacks, and the best peach tea in the United States. Just being around others with like experiences, needs and challenges seems to lift the spirit.

Kindred spirits gather for treatment, but they also share experiences and swap stories about how they are making it through treatments. Some have happy things to tell while others may not be so fortunate and just need a hand to hold.

In short, West Clinic is a place of respite, of encouragement, of a gathering of like minds and hearts with a shared challenge called cancer. This chapter is about some very special people.

Volunteer Jean Reed with Director Gigi Lee and Lorna Mize

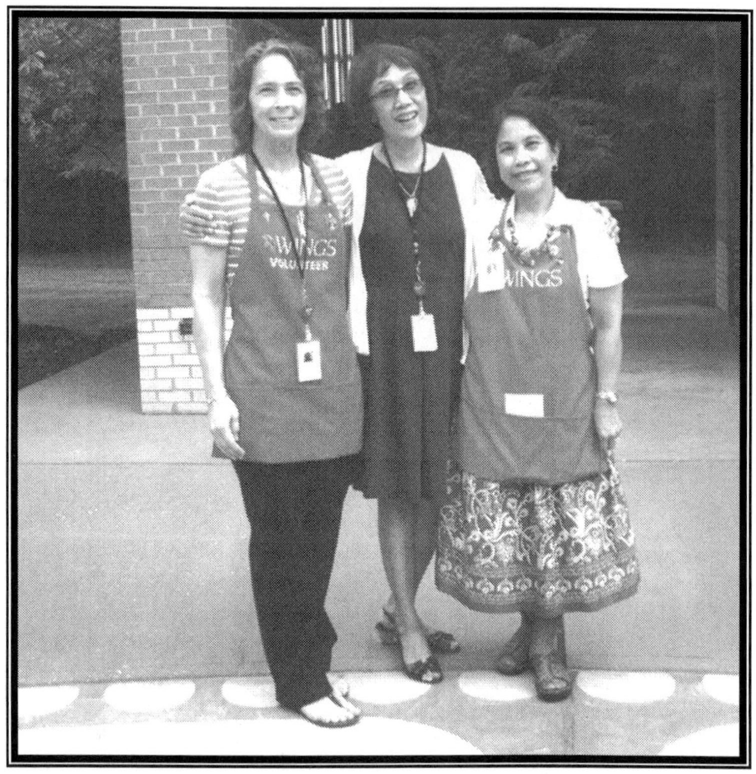

We, as patients, are kindly and professionally served by members of the Wings organization who volunteer their time just to be able to minister to patients. They hand out blankets, teddy bears, hats, treats, and smiles galore, and they always have friendly, happy words for the patients.

Let me take this opportunity to introduce you to the two ladies that allowed the above picture to be taken with Gigi Lee for our book.

First, the lovely lady on the far left is Jean Reed, a fifty-two year-old wife and mother of a twenty-seven year-old son, a daughter who is twenty-five, and "Granny" to a precious grandson. She came across as a spunky fighter who is no stranger to being knocked down and getting back up.

Her story is close to my heart in that her cancer was the same as mine, Squamous cell carcinoma that emanated from her tonsil area where a tumor had formed.

Jean. Painful symptoms had prompted me to seek medical attention and those complaints were diagnosed as tonsillitis and an ear-ache. Antibiotics were prescribed, the symptoms were reduced, but I was back for more tests in June, for which I received the same diagnosis and treatment.

Mike. In November, Jean's ENT specialist ordered a CT scan that disclosed a tumor on her tonsil. A subsequent biopsy indicated Squamous cell carcinoma with a positive reading for HPV virus that seems to be the culprit in this type cancer. That was in January 2013.

Jean. When I was diagnosed and heard the "you've got cancer," proclamation, I was scared to death. I asked God, "why me?" I felt guilty about having smoked at one time; wondered what would happen next and would I die? Would I live? And then I simply disconnected from normalcy and reality –I, as they say, zoned out.

Mike. What Jean said next summed up the next few months of her life.

Jean. I took a quick trip to and through Hell and back. I was fortunate in many ways in that my treatments lasted only two months. I had two rounds of three kinds of chemo to prep me for surgery. Although my first doctor said I wouldn't lose my hair, I did, and I became a card carrying member of the "Bald is Beautiful Club.

After the treatments, I underwent surgery to remove half my tonsils and all the lymph nodes from the side of my neck area. The surgery was extensive and deep, and I have a six-inch scar to remind me of the process that left me with more scarring around the area of my tonsil and inside my cheek. To this day I have trouble swallowing.

The surgical process that removed a large mass at the base of my tongue didn't cause me a great deal of pain, but it did leave me unable to open my mouth very wide due to it being held wide open for so long during the surgery.

It required weeks of effort and exercise for my mouth to return to normal. What I call pins and needles pain along the side of my tongue remains to this day. But I am cancer free, with just a few trappings of the treatment remaining for me to remember my journey.

I remember one evening after taking a shower, I found myself looking in my bathroom mirror. Instead of my own reflection, I saw my fifty-six year-old mother who had died of lung cancer when I was twenty-seven. That was the type of in-and-out-of-reality experience I had at times.

As uncomfortable as my experience was, it was bearable; and the outcome was worth the discomfort. I had experienced a number of hard knocks before my diagnosis. Cancer became another challenge that would contribute to me becoming a better person in several ways.

I began focusing on others rather than myself. I used my discomfort as a base and to establish credibility and acceptance in order to help others, and to develop and provide empathy where it is needed to give hope to patients who needed it.

My best friend during treatment was my three year-old female Chocolate Lab, Bailey. We would walk at the dog park close to our home, and she just seemed to understand my condition.

Often times Bailey would come to me; place her head on my upper leg and just be there. This was my therapy, and I found my dog to be more sympathetic than some of the doctors I encountered.

After treatment, I found that I had developed a desire to be with the patients at West Clinic and to do what I could to lift them up from where they were. What I found was that they lifted me up as I was ministering to them. What I sent out from my spirit to them came back to me many times over. That's really why I continue as a volunteer for Wings.

I won't leave you with the assumption that all is roses and I no longer fight the demons of after treatment woes. I am being treated for depression and anxiety that are my constant companions. I push through them in order to function. But push through them I do.

I am thankful to be alive and cancer free. Cancer has put me in touch with my own mortality and I realize that life is fragile and that we are not guaranteed tomorrow, next week, or next year. So I am making the most of what I have today.

I would not have chosen this path to walk, nor would I have chosen the terrible things that I endured to be free of a powerful and lethal enemy. I do believe, however, that I am a better person for having been there, for having experienced the many aspects of the emotional, physical, and spiritual challenges of cancer, and coming out the other side.

Life doesn't return to normal after cancer treatments. That pre-cancer person or "normal" no longer exists. I am learning to embrace my new "normal." I know that by the grace of God and with my supporting family, friends and dog, I will get thru it.

§

Mike. The beautiful lady on the far right is from the Philippines, is married, fifty-eight years old, and has been a Wings volunteer for four years.

She is technically educated and highly astute as a food scientist with several major food companies over her career. She was responsible for the formulation and production of major brands of human and pet food products.

During the interview, Lorna Mize came across as analytical and savvy in the world of science and technology. She is also an obviously healthy and disciplined person.

In December 2005, Lorna explained that she began to feel tired and ran a low-grade fever and began to feel full too early when eating, which is called early satiety. When she began being short of breath, she became concerned to the point of seeking medical help. With that, I will let Lorna tell her story.

§

Lorna. A physical examination by my doctor disclosed that my spleen had enlarged, and he referred me to a surgeon for possible removal. He sent me for a CT scan which confirmed that my spleen had enlarged sufficiently to press against my left lung causing the shortness of breath. A lymphoproliferative disorder including lymphoma was highly suggested by the radiologist.

The surgeon had received a copy of the scan results. While she was briefing me about the surgery she began a telephone conversation with an oncologist. I overheard terms such as 'the enlarged spleen will respond to chemo.' After the phone conversation, she told me, 'Unfortunately you have lymphoma.' These words blew my mind.

I drove home by myself in complete shock not knowing what to do. That was when I began to question God, went through shock, and then on to grieving over my circumstances.

In January 2006, the surgeon performed excisional lymph node and bone marrow core biopsies. The diagnosis was non-Hodgkin, B-cell, stage four, grade three, follicular lymphoma.

My medical team sent me to a cancer clinic where I entered what is called a phase three clinical study from which the protocols for my treatment were established. I would receive a cocktail of chemotherapy drugs and monoclonal anti-bodies.

Side effects of the treatment were fairly standard. Hair loss, weakness, constipation, metallic taste in my mouth, peripheral neuropathy, moderate weight gain but it was not more than I could handle, and it did not put me down as some I have seen.

I tolerated the treatment sufficiently well in that I was able to work at my job throughout the process. I'll never forget the valuable advice I was given by one of my professional care givers. 'Treat your energy like a bank. Make deposits and withdrawals only when necessary.' How true that was, and I found it to be invaluable in getting through each day.

Six cycles of chemo and four of monoclonal anti-bodies were administered, after which the scans indicated that I was cancer-free.

In March 2011, I became a Wings volunteer. I had seen God's sovereignty in my circumstances and was thankful that my life had been spared. I earnestly desire to give Him all the glory in carrying me through it all.

As a Wings volunteer, I am sensitive to the varying levels of religious beliefs and sensitivities. Being a Christian and practicing Nazarene, I will share Jesus every chance I get. But this is not an approach for everyone who comes to West Clinic. There are, however, some constants that I feel free to share with everyone.

My message to any patient is that they are in a wonderful place with the best care available. West Clinic is a high-tech organization with the latest monitoring devices that remains current with the latest discoveries and breakthroughs. This is a place of hope and healing.

I am proud to be a part of our organization, and I firmly believe there is no better place to receive the latest available care for cancer patients. I am thankful for West Clinic and for Wings Cancer Foundation that gave me a chance to serve.

§

Mike. I discovered some interesting facts about the volunteers and programs offered, such as support groups, exercise and strength programs, nutrition counseling, and holistic therapies.

One of the more interesting concepts, espoused one of the members is that "*hugs heal.*" That has become the program motto, and hugs reign supreme and run free.

What Wings volunteers do best is offer hope and courage; a touch, a hug, a smile. Kind words from a seasoned cancer survivor or care giver combine with a pleasant countenance to make powerful medicine.

Those folks know what it means to sit in a waiting room or be strapped to an IV in the infusion room itself. They know the look, the appearance and blank stares of certain desperate folks. They make a huge difference in the visit for treatment, scans, or doctor's follow-ups. They are true angels of love and mercy.

What I found out about the Wings volunteers is that each one is either a cancer survivor or care giver. After the patients finish their treatments and regain their strength and stamina, they can volunteer to serve and encourage the approximately 300 patients a day that are seen at West Clinic Humphreys Center.

I lifted the following information from the Wings website, www.wingscancerfoundation.org, and I strongly recommend that you access, read, and support their cause. They significantly helped me through a very trying ordeal.

Wings Cancer Foundation is a 501c3 non-profit whose purpose is to meet the physical, emotional and spiritual needs of cancer patients and their families. When a diagnosis of cancer turns lives upside down, Wings programs and services can help, and no one is ever charged.

Like the word wings implies in nature, Wings Cancer Foundation is all about support through an essential relationship. Everything we do is designed to foster hope, educate and provide support to cancer patients and families - all at no cost. *With years of practical experience, and in some cases cancer survival, our team of professionals and network of services focuses on meeting the needs of those fighting cancer.*

The person who may be one of the most recognizable is a lady who was there for Judy when she was being treated, and is still there to help me, belongs to Gigi Lee, the lady in the center of the above picture.

A background in staff development and teaching adults prepared her to train, educate, and support two hundred plus volunteers in East Memphis, Midtown, and Southaven, Mississippi. I remember her wise words.

Gigi. Delivering compassionate care from one cancer survivor to another is something a teacher cannot teach a student. Volunteers serve because they are passionate about building strong human connections; these relationships sustain the foundation of survivorship and well-being. And it is my utmost privilege and honor to witness this gift of giving. In this sense, I am the student, and volunteers are my teachers.

Mike. Gigi retired the last of October of 2014, and we will miss her a great deal.

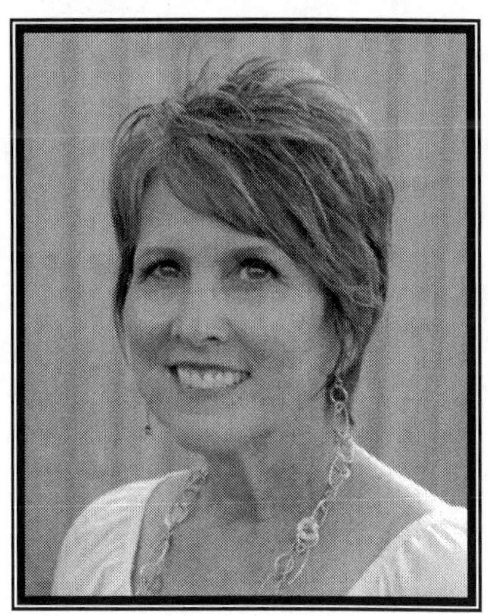

Mike. As a Southern Baptist, I haven't worked with many female ministers; God really changed that. I'll say more about how Sharon is shaping my personal and ministerial life later.

Chaplain Sharon Herlihy is responsible for the Wings Pastoral Care Ministry and is our mentor in cancer support. This is the lady that in what may have been one of my darkest hours, in the infusion room, dropped to her knees and prayed for me with about thirty patients and their family members looking on. She joined the Wings staff in June 2011, bringing spiritual care and support to patients and their families through weekly prayer circles, group support, and individual encouragement.

Sharon. I am an ordained minister with the Assemblies of God. My greatest desire is to help people find hope in the midst of their cancer journey, regardless of their particular denomination or faith background. Sometimes, ministry simply means listening with my whole heart. People often just need a listening ear more than anything else. I am available by phone, email or by appointment at each Wings location.

§

Mike. Our home church, Bartlett Hills Baptist Church has initiated a cancer support group that is open to the entire community. We needed all the support, assets, educational materials, and expertise that we could get.

As we began this new ministry, we discovered that in many ways it was a new concept in church and community interactions. We felt it wise to employ all the available, successful, professional and available resources at our disposal.

There are few cancer support groups in the United States, hosted by churches. Most are tied to Cancer Treatment organizations and even then, they are too few to reach the myriad and diverse cancer survivors and care givers that need help and encouragement. Wings Cancer Foundation graciously offered to help us organize and initiate the Faith in the Face of Cancer group that is meeting monthly and welcomes anyone who desires to attend. We'll talk about this a bit more at the end of the book.

§

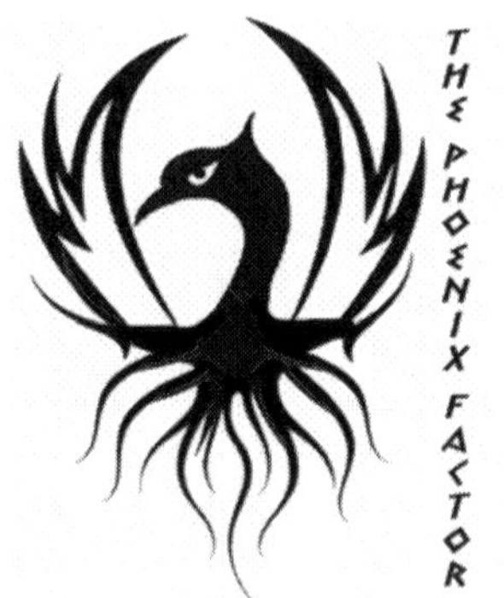

This chapter has been about people helping people through difficult times. Volunteers, fellow cancer survivors, care givers, and organizations standing by to serve.

Cancer is tough, and it takes a heavy toll, but we are not alone. There are those who have enough love to share, and they do it unselfishly, unrelenting, and willingly.

§§§

Chapter Seven

A Word about the Disease

What is Cancer? Cancer is a harsh and devastating disease characterized by out-of-control cell growth. There are well over a hundred major different types of cancer, and each is classified by the type of cell that is initially affected and where it originates. Actually, there are between two and three hundred types of cancer if one cares to define them as to specifics.

Cancer harms the body when damaged cells divide uncontrollably and form lumps or masses of tissue called tumors. Leukemia, on the other hand, prohibits normal blood function by abnormal cell division in the blood stream.

Tumors can grow and interfere with the digestive, nervous, and circulatory systems and they can release hormones that alter body functions. Tumors that stay in one spot and demonstrate limited growth are generally considered to be *benign.* The spreading of these abnormal cells or tumors is called *metastasis.*

Cancer is ultimately the result of cells that uncontrollably grow and do not die. Normal cells in the body follow an orderly path of growth, division, and death.

Programmed cell death is called *apoptosis,* and when this process breaks down, cancer begins to form. Unlike regular cells, cancer cells do not experience programmatic death, and instead they continue to grow and divide. This leads to a mass of abnormal cells that grows out of control.

We have all heard about the stages of cancer. There are actually five stages, but Stage 0 counts as one, so there is actually no Stage V Cancer. Simply put,

- Stage 0, or *carcinoma in situ* is called very early cancer.
- Stage I means that cancer cells have involved the primary site from which the cancer will derive its name.
- Stage II, indicates that it has spread to nearby areas.
- Stage III, cancer has spread throughout the nearby area.
- Stage IV, it has spread to other parts of the body.

Cancer is the number two killer in America currently, just after heart disease as number one. About one in three Americans have been or will be diagnosed with cancer. It has affected roughly seven and a third million people that are currently living in the United States.

Cancer kills over fifteen hundred U.S. citizens every day, and nearly six hundred thousand Americans in a single year; that number is rising. From all estimates, it appears that about forty to fifty percent of all humans have cancer.

That's all the science we need for our purpose. This book is a layperson's approach to a very technical, medical issue. For the authors to venture into the specific field of oncology would prove disastrous.

§

There is one area of West Cancer Clinic that brings together, on a recurring basis, most of the three hundred patients a day that are seen there.

The patients are introduced to this room early on, visit it on a regular basis, get to know it well, and find that it becomes a social as well as a treatment area for some.

The infusion room has more return customers than does any other place in the clinic with the exception of the phlebotomy lab. The *phlebe lab* is where blood is taken for testing, and patients are hooked up with the Huber needle connectors through which infusions and various scan dyes are injected into the body.

By the time I first visited West Clinic, I had already been diagnosed, prepped, educated, and had chemotherapy begun as a treatment in the hospital.

One visit with the oncologist and I was set up for the infusion room and the side effects of chemotherapy. So, one might say that the infusion room was my mainstay for cancer treatment, and the professionals that run and serve in the room were very much responsible for my positive attitude during the treatments.

If you visit the infusion room at the Humphreys West Clinic, you will find about thirty-five chairs and five beds used to infuse medications into patients requiring blood, injections, iron deficiency solutions, auto immune medications, and more.

There are ten nurses and nurse practitioners that provide services to the patients five and a half days a week. Mostly, the chairs are full with family members or friends sitting next to the patient waiting to transport them home after treatment.

The first thing that struck me as unusual about being cared for in this large and busy room was that I was treated as an important human being, and not just a number or patient.

Patience and kindness earmarked each of the nurses and nurse practioners that served my needs. They were never short with me or seemed to be in too much of a hurry to take special care of me. There were times when there were a lot of patients requiring a lot of interaction, but there was always time for me.

Questions are always answered or the answer is researched and provided when the information is sure to be correct. The nurses never assume the role of the doctor, but there are very few times that they defer to the primary oncologist.

The crew goes out of its way to provide complete treatment, informative feedback, referrals to other service providers in the clinic, and understand the comfort and emotional needs of a cancer patient. These medical care-givers became my friends. They are my heroes, and they are held in very high esteem by me and thousands of others.

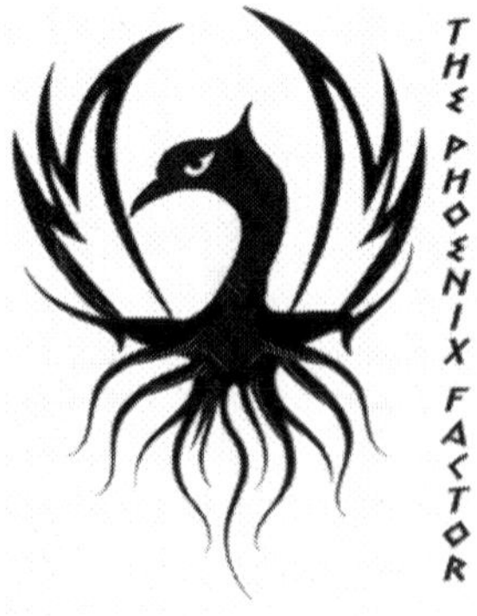

The more we know about cancer, the more we realize how it will one day be defeated by a team effort –a team the size of the whole realm of medical science. The team that cared for me is one of thousands like it. Thank God for the professionals who care enough to fight the good fight.

§§§

Chapter Eight

Paws for Distraction – Jo Anne Fusco, Kicker and Boss

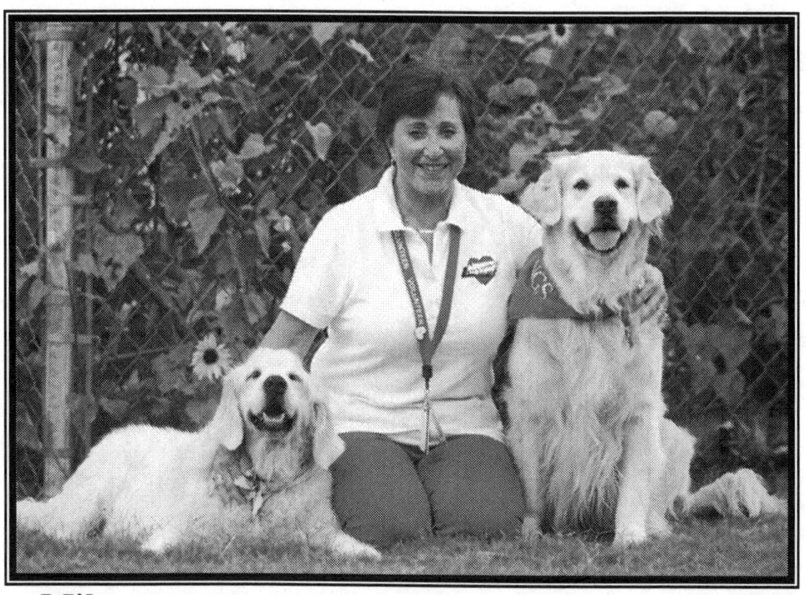

Mike. Before returning to what I call the moan and groan part of our book, I want to include some nice words about my favorite team of encouragers.

You might find the next chapter a bit unusual, in that it incorporates an unexpected surprise amid the otherwise somewhat bleak picture we are painting so far.

I think that I enjoyed working on this section of the book more than any others. My son, wife, grandchildren and I all went for a photo shoot with the subjects of the next chapter, and walked away happy and glad that there are such unusual blessings in the world of therapy and rehabilitation.

Oftentimes, cancer patients sink so low in their strength, outlook, frustration, pain and discomfort, that no amount of words really helps, and prayer, although powerful and welcome, doesn't bring immediate relief.

There is a team of magic and wonder weavers that never fails to bring smiles and sighs, and helps the patient to forget for a few moments who they are and why they are at West Clinic.

§

I was in the waiting area outside the infusion room at West Cancer Treatment Center, contemplating my woes, my last infusion, and the treatment I was about to receive.

I had just been served some of the best peach iced tea I'd ever had by a Wings volunteer, who herself was a cancer survivor. All of a sudden the room was filled with the electricity of excited people focusing on something special.

That's when I first encountered a real; honest to goodness blessing right in the middle of a bunch of folks who needed a soul boost.

I first felt a presence, and then I noticed two big beautiful eyes, long blondish hair, and big black nose. I learned that this thirteen year-old, golden retriever's name was *Kicker*.

As soon as I extended a welcome to Kicker, he placed his head on my knee and just sat there letting the love pour out. His handshakes brought squeals of delight from the ladies and smiles from the men.

Kicker's handler and owner is *Jo-Jo*, or Jo Anne Fusco. We learned that Kicker is himself a three-year cancer survivor, so he has been there, done that, and has the tee-shirt.

That was my first encounter with therapy dogs, and all 65 pounds of this canine were loaded with warm fuzzies, affection, and a strange but real sensation that he knows the ropes, feels the needs, and gives everything he has to anyone who wants it.

Kicker is not what may be called a civilian, police or military service dog, such as a cadaver, explosive sniffing, rescue, or drug dog. Neither is he used as a blind lead dog, or assistant to the deaf, seizure or diabetic crisis detection.

Kicker is a therapy dog whose only job is to bring comfort by putting people at ease and allow hurting, anxious, frightened patients to hug and pet them.

I found that one of the most fascinating tasks for Kicker and his non-biological canine brother *Boss*, a seven year-old golden retriever, is sitting with kids who could use a little encouragement to read aloud. These dogs don't negatively react to stuttering or stumbling over words, and they do not become impatient.

Usually, the only dog one will see in restaurants, or other semi private public areas are the blind lead, and service dogs. Under the Federal Americans with Disabilities Act these dogs can go anywhere their masters can.

There are about fifty such dogs in the Memphis area. Hopefully there will be more in the future. So restaurants, planes, public places that do not allow dogs will not allow a therapy animal.

§

Jo-Jo. Therapy dogs are allowed with their handler and identification into places that have invited them and with whom they are working.

So Boss and Kicker go to Saint Jude's, but only on Tuesdays at 9:30 a.m. when it's *doggie times*. I am only allowed one dog at a time in keeping with the rules of Therapy Dogs Incorporated.

Kicker, Boss and I are a registered team that has been tested, evaluated and re-evaluated. We go to West Cancer Clinic, Methodist Hospital, Memphis International Airport, The Oral School for the Deaf, the Exceptional Foundation for Special Needs Individuals, where I am the Executive Director, Hospice, and we are pursuing working with children with the Child Advocacy Center.

I started West Tennessee Therapy Dogs, and we presently have over thirty-five members. All of our members are tested through a national organization such as Therapy dogs, Incorporated.

§

Mike. Jo-Jo explained to me that just because dogs may be gentle or mild mannered, doesn't make them good therapy dogs. The canine must be trained, disciplined, certified, and manifest calm under duress, in a crowd. They must not become spooked by squeals, wheel chairs, walkers, or pats that might be a little too hard.

I became so impressed with Jo-Jo and her dogs' kind and patient service that we wanted to tell about them in this book. They were instrumental in bringing me peace and distraction during the six months of treatment. They were real stress dissipaters; and it has been proven that a lack of bad stress accelerates healing.

As she said earlier, Jo-Jo, Kicker, and Boss frequent nursing homes, day care facilities, children's hospitals, cancer treatment facilities and any other care giving facility that might request their services.

I am one thankful patient to have benefitted from their special gift to those in need of something that cannot be bought.

Folks with Alzheimer's disease, dementia; those who are dying, and frightened; or confused hurting children, and the elderly are all potential recipients for the unique and special kind of love that is provided by one lady and two dogs. What they do could be called, magical, wonderful, spiritual, powerful, and amazingly nice.

I have been a Sunday School teacher, deacon, and sort of a lay minister for over forty-five years. I am a big proponent of random acts of kindness and being a blessing to others. I have seen first hand the difference these kindnesses make in the lives of the recipients.

Jo-Jo related that she was reared to practice what our Jewish brethren call the giving of mitzvahs, or acts of kindness –she feels that these are ways of giving back some of one's many blessings. What is important to know here is that this mitzvah would not happen if it were not for the Jo-Jo's, Kickers, and Bosses of the world.

Now you need to grab a hankie as I relate the heart-warming part of this tale of two tails. I sometimes feel old, broken up, used up, fed up, and pretty shallow with most of my life being behind me now. These three team members have caused me to rethink my situation.

When Jo-Jo and Kicker enter the presence of a chemo or radiation patient, she tells them of Kicker's unique qualifications to serve their needs and bring them some comfort.

Three years ago, Kicker was diagnosed with non-Hodgkin's lymphoma and underwent extensive chemotherapy –now, I can relate to that.

The treatment saved his life, but weakened his back legs, causing him to lose his footing on hard bare floors without carpet –I can relate to that also.

Kicker is no longer the spry, nimble pooch that walked with an energetic bustle as he once did. Now he is quiet, passive, slow, deliberate, and cautious in his walk. He was knocked down pretty hard, but he rose again to serve not only his master, but anyone needing his love –I can sure relate to that too.

But, like Kicker, I do have a lot more credibility with other cancer patients when they find out that I am a survivor and have been where they are.

Patients are invited by Jo-Jo to pet, touch, even hug or shake hands (or paws) with Kicker, or maybe just look at him; that has a calming effect. When all is said and done, hand sanitizer is provided to the patients just to make sure no germs are transferred. Not many are the times that Jo-Jo and friends depart without a lot of smiles and verbal goodbyes.

There are some people who like dogs, some who don't, others prefer not to be bothered, but most are in desperate need of help in getting through what may be the toughest time of their life. As one lady put it, Kicker put a smile on her face and for just a few minutes helped her forget why she was in the infusion room with an IV in her arm.

Jo-Jo is a trained, experienced, savvy and tender-hearted care giver and reads patients very well as to their acceptance of Kicker or Boss. The older and more experienced Kicker seems to have a radar or gauge to let him know how much attention someone needs and when their cup begins to run over. It's uncanny how he senses tension, desperation, sadness, hopelessness, and frustration.

We'd be more than negligent if we didn't add here how to contact Jo-Jo to request her services. Simply send an e-mail to fuscojo@aol.com

That about sums it up for my first experience with therapy dogs. Selfless, loyal, loving, and devoted animals, with large beautiful eyes, long blondish hair, and black noses.

Judy and I are dog lovers, and we can attest to the pain we experienced as we had our Sheltie euthanized when he was seventeen years old –very old for a pooch.

As pet owners, people have the privilege of providing shelter, food, recreation, medical services, grooming, love, and all the amenities they can lavish on their four-footed family member.

They also have the sacred and sometimes overwhelmingly hard responsibility for making decisions that the pets cannot make for themselves. When to stop a life is just about as sacred as it gets; when it is the life of your beloved family member, that's about as difficult as it gets.

Oh that hurt our hearts. *Yago* couldn't walk as well anymore; he was deaf; his back legs would lock up; He had lost some teeth, and he had cataracts.

Selfishly, we kept him around because he gave us so much. Sometimes I think I can hear his bark in the distance. I have even stopped what I was doing to look up and strain my ears. I am sure it is only my imagination.

I am so glad that Kicker kicked his cancer. I can honestly empathize with how Jo-Jo must have felt as she dealt with the possibility of Kicker succumbing to his disease.

Kicker and Boss give so much to others –they are a real inspiration and proved that they will be man's best friend until the very end –which I hope is a long, long time from now.

Kicker and Boss…take a bow…wow!

§

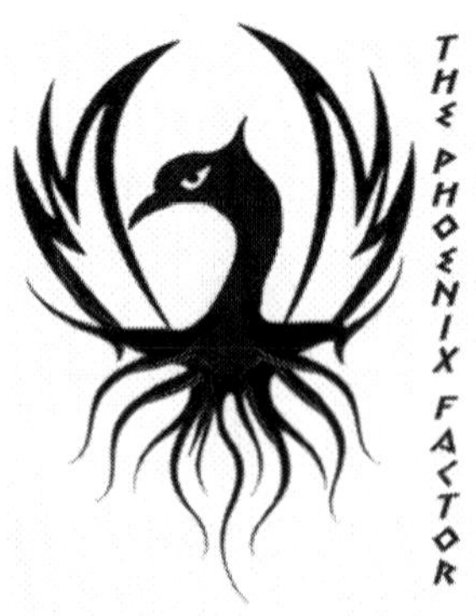

"Man's Best Friend" didn't earn that title by not being sensitive to his master's feelings. Kicker and Boss are marvelous to watch and I always came away overwhelmed by what I observed. Dogs are far more discerning, intuitive, and aware of their surroundings than we give them credit for.

§§§

Chapter Nine

The Challenges of Chemo

When I returned home from the hospital, I was a bit over three weeks into my treatment, and was very much under the influence of chemotherapy, blood thinners, and the chills that come from newly acquired baldness (NAB) as I call it.

When you see cancer patients wearing scarves, hats, ski caps, and those nifty looking English driving, casual grey herringbone wool ivy caps that look like they came from Jolly Old England, it may be because they are cold.

Hair is an insulator and when it disappears; your body doesn't know how to react, so it allows you to freeze. Of course some folks do feel self conscious about being bald and want to cover the source of their embarrassment –bald isn't always beautiful.

At this point, I am still being needle pricked for infusions because I do not have my port yet. My arms are black and blue, I have bruises where I struck objects while trying to walk, my head looks like one of those old cabbage patch dolls with just a few strands of hair here and there –ugly, ugly, ugly.

Our friend Sheila Harrell is a hair cutter, par excellence, and agreed to give me a buzz cut to get ride of the few hairs that remained. She had to be very careful not to nick me, cut me, scratch me, or scrape me, because I might bleed profusely.

By now I have lost my taste and in its place developed a serious revulsion for the texture or smell of solid food. I could not stand to chew anything, smells nauseated me, and it was all I could do to drink a famous nutritional liquid that is used in medical feeding tubes for patients that can't swallow. I know this sounds a bit far out, but it is the truth. I tried to bite off and chew the end of a pretzel; I almost threw up and I did gag.

I must admit, I did look a bit like Mister Clean with my new bald head. That is where the similarity stopped, because I didn't have his muscles and physique. What remained after a buzz cut fell out over the next few weeks, and I became polished, shiny, slick, and bald.

§

I commandeered my beloved's comfortable recliner where I remained for nine months. It became my roost, my friend, my sanctuary, and my comfort.

A dear friend; a lady for whom I had done a favor once, had hand made a neat blanket for me a while back, and it became my inseparable warmer and security blanket –thanks Barbara.

I could remain still and watch television, do a bit of social media surfing, and read until my eyes became weak and knocked out that pleasure. But at least I was home, except for my trips to the clinic and hospital.

My treatments consisted of fluids, one chemo, and another, then a pump which was attached that dripped another chemo over a four day period.

After being wired up with the pump for several days and watching the monitor to see when the tank was empty, I returned to the clinic to have the pump removed and was then sent home for three weeks, or so.

On day three, the treatment began to knock my socks off and I became nauseous, dizzy, weak, constipated, and lethargic to the point of curling up into the fetal position and not moving for days –trust Jesus.

§

E-mails, cards, calls, gifts, food, and visits are the mainstay of getting through recovery and undergoing surgery or treatment. But even vital things that are as positive and encouraging as these can become somewhat trying.

Too much of a good thing becomes not a good thing. Too many, too often, too long, or even favors done at the wrong time can be counter-productive. The wrong things being said and failing to consider just how sick, tired, and weary the patient is can be irritating and wearing on a friendship.

This may sound strange, but no matter how sick someone might be, they usually still feel compelled to entertain their visitors.

I need to interject a thought here. During the nine months of my own personal agony, my beloved was going through her own stress, frustration, worry, fears, weakness, fatigue, overwork, under-play, and need for some kind of positive diversion.

The spouse needs consideration during these ordeals, and I promise that invitations to lunch, a movie, shopping, or anything that a lady or man likes to do are welcome, if there is an offer to sit with the patient while she or avails herself of the kind offer.

There were several folks who did this for us. Some even took me for my infusions and gave Judy a break. Infusions can last three to four hours.

Thankfully, we have friends who very considerately provided these diversions without being asked. And to settle a question that might arise here, there was no way I could convince Judy to go out and leave me by myself. It just wasn't going to happen.

As a very sick, weak, mentally exhausted and uncomfortable person, many times I did not want to talk on the telephone, conduct two way conversations that reiterated my condition, or even try to be nice to people –that made me feel guilty. Please allow a bit of time here for some *grossity* as I call it.

There were times, many times, when I had gastro-intestinal issues that caused great discomfort. Failure to eliminate can make a person pray for comfort, but entertaining guests becomes very low on a list of priorities.

During these times, the mature and thoughtful visitor will chat more with the spouse less with the patient. Guests should be forgiving and cooperative, and not be put out if the patient doesn't respond to them or meet social expectations. Most folks are sensitive to these issues and graciously cooperate.

There were times in the hospital when I was using a urinal that I had to ask visitors to leave while I relieved myself. A good rule of thumb is what I learned as a young deacon about making hospital visits –15 minutes. If the patient asks you to stay a bit longer, be receptive, but try not to establish the value of a visit by the length of your stay.

Here is a nugget of gold or precious jewel worth keeping. *Sometimes, especially men would like just a bit of alone time, a bit of privacy, and a quiet moment or two.*

When you consider all the medical staff interventions, visitors, phone calls, tests, medications, meals, and room services, there isn't much time left over for privacy or rest.

§

Now that we have those somewhat negative issues out of the way, let me say that cancer patients are somewhat unique in that they are being systematically poisoned.

Chemotherapy is a lot like the treatment for amoebae that invade the body and cause dysentery. We used to call it Montezuma's revenge for your visit south of the border.

In the past, arsenic was used to kill the parasites. Arsenic, like chemo, is poison and can on its own kill the patient. More advanced treatments are now available, but the basic design is the same –kill the parasites or malformed cells.

Amebiasis (amebic dysentery) is a parasitic infection of the large intestine or liver common in developing countries. It takes a highly trained and informed specialist to identify, diagnose, prescribe, and regulate chemotherapy so that it will cure rather than kill.

So the cancer patient, (me for example), is going to be very sick and manifest the same symptoms as a poisoning victim. Organs are affected, so are glands, intestines, and everything in the body, because chemotherapy circulates with the blood and goes where the blood goes. Let me provide a graphic example of how far reaching it is.

I have always battled toenail fungus, like most people. In the eighth month of treatment, we went to our home in Branson, where I decided to trim my toenails. Guess what? Every toenail fell off in my hand. The chemo had killed the fungus that was holding the nail in place.

My fingernails turned pale and became brittle and ridged. There were several mole-like spots on my body that disappeared. I did not shave for six months –no beard.

My creatinine levels have not returned to normal and I always have a strange taste in my mouth, as if I need to brush my teeth – which I do.

§

As I had more treatments, each one built on the others and built up chemo levels in my body seeking out the cells which didn't belong and destroying them.

That's what chemo is all about. In the process, I had to be monitored for dehydration, heart rate, blood pressure, oxygenation levels, blood count, and several other blood levels that indicated normal or abnormal functioning of organs and glands. Sugar levels are important as are the dozens of other test indicators.

Mix this with steroids that string you out like a violin and rob you of sleep, fill you with a strange pseudo energy that you can use for just about nothing, and keeps you alert to the other not-so -great things that are happening to you. What good are steroids?

The doctor says they are good for what ails you, if they don't drive you over the edge.

There were times after each treatment when I experienced high fever complete with chills –I hate chills. That produced delirium. This is important, and I want to take a moment to share the results of my research into it.

Delirium is a condition in which I became unfocused and confused. There are different causes for this condition, fever is one. A fever can cause delirium when elevated body temperatures interfere with metabolism.

For a fever to cause delirium, the body must reach a temperature of at least 105 degrees Fahrenheit or more in most cases. Fevers of 104 degrees Fahrenheit or lower typically do not cause the condition.

Like fever, delirium is a symptom of an underlying cause. Delirium can also be caused by poison, brain injury, and withdrawal from certain addictive substances, severe shock, and diseases.

Delirium accompanied by high fever can indicate infectious disease or any number of conditions of the body. They are however, typically not the only symptoms of a condition or disease.

High fevers and delirium may be present, as well as seizures. Again, seizures associated with high fevers are considered acute and may or may not be a sign of another problem.

Typically, both delirium and seizures associated with excessively high fevers dissipate when the fever breaks. There is always the potential for complications with a high fever.

Here is the interesting part of these experiences. I was so out of it that I didn't know enough to call for help. I remember when my bed, alarm clock, light, and bottle of water became a cacophonous synergy of out of synch computer functions.

I could not in my head, get them to work right. I had images of computer screens, flowing water, digital clock numbers, all melding with my bed to where I was inside a computer trying to get warm.

Then the fever would break and blessed sleep would come. On the humorous side, my youngest granddaughter kids me about not being right. After those dreams or hallucinations or delirium episodes, I wasn't so sure she was kidding.

I remember one very scary night when I had a bad episode, got violently nauseous, threw up through my trach into a pan we kept by my side, got chocolate nutrition drink mixed with blood and mucous all over myself, and then could not call for help to Judy who was sleeping on the couch.

To make matters worse, my coordination was non-existent at that point, and I tilted the pan spilling the contents of the regurgitation all over my head and face. Now we had a stained pillow, bed sheets, and a slimy Mike –trust Jesus.

Showers were always fun and often ended in my passing out or nearly doing so. I experienced a strange event that I have yet to find a doctor who could tell me what it was or why I was seeing the light at the end of the tunnel. The same light that you hear people say they see during near death experiences.

My cardiologist suspected that the hot water that cascaded over my bald head was stimulating the brain or arteries causing the phenomenon.

As I shampooed my head and rinsed it with very warm water, a light that appeared to be in the shape of an eye began to take form and become brighter. It continued until I collapsed.

I learned to watch and not allow it to get to the brightest passing out stage. I still see the image but it doesn't get as bright as it used to. I have my own suspicions about the origin, but I am not a doctor and I do not want to plant any notions in your head.

One last shower related oddity was that my bald head would sting and itch and burn from the shampoo. I would scratch an itch, and it would swell into a large knot. I would have them in four or five places on my scalp making me look like an alien out of a Sci-Fi movie.

§

With apologies to Joan Rivers, can we talk? I am going to try to describe what and who I was when I hit bottom and before I began the trip back to what I call normalcy. That for me is a lot different than it was (BC) before cancer.

As a writer, I have become hundreds of characters for my novels by crawling into their skin and thinking like they think. I have been a man, woman, child, teenager, serial killer, robber, thief, addict, murderer, terrorist, priest, preacher, cop, deviate, psycho, schizo, sociopath, military sniper, diver, and have thoroughly probed the criminal mind.

But I had never been a cancer patient before. I couldn't close the page and walk away from this character. The motivator for who I had become was coursing through my veins and trying to kill abnormal cells without killing me. It was a delicate balancing act that my oncologist closely monitored.

§

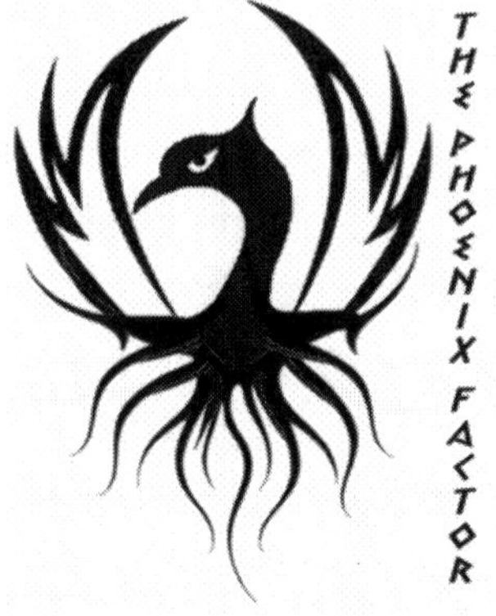

I have learned from Cancer that we often become stagnated in maturing once we reach a certain age and become comfortable with our regimen, schedule, recreation, profession, faith related matters, and social life.

Cancer has a way of adding dimensions to our life and thus helps us to expand our mind and spirit into areas we would not have chosen for ourselves, but prove to be positive additions to our character.

§§§

Chapter Ten

Overcoming

This will be one of the more important chapters in the book. I am going to talk about making the best out of the worst situation, extracting good from bad, and making lemonade out of the lemons of life.

After four hospitalizations, perhaps a hundred units of fluids, five rounds of triple chemo, surgery, biopsies, starvation, 130 pounds of weight-loss, and no solid food for nine months, I was what you might call, a mess.

God loves messes. In fact, you almost have to be a mess before you can truly call out to Him and invite Jesus into your heart. But how can He straighten out my mess?

First off, can we agree that humans, especially Americans have a high standard of living they try very hard to achieve? It consists of having as many modern gadgets as they can buy, a nice home with heat and air, all they can eat, and comforts of every imaginable sort.

We sometimes want people to do our hair, nails, and teeth, clean our houses, wash our cars, mow our lawns, and bring us our food and drink while we watch sports, do the social media thing, or play internet games.

Most everyone wants money in the bank, a secure retirement, health insurance, credit cards, a good church, lots of friends, and children and grandchildren who make us proud –then comes cancer.

Let's take away just about every creature comfort, because mostly you won't enjoy them anymore. Take away your mobility, because you don't want to go anywhere. Take away the primping, prepping, and playing, because none of it is any fun anymore.

You have no hair to coif, no nails to manicure, toenails to pedicure, teeth to clean or drill, and no appetite for food of any kind.

Add to the above, extreme fatigue, weakness, coordination, bowel issues, and the infernal feeling of ant stings that come when you get out in the sun and heat, the odors, the trach messes, the irritations, and sleepless nights, and you have me and many other cancer patients.

Now let me think; the title of this book is Thank You God for Cancer. At this point, you may just think that is a bit far out and even harder to reach; not really –trust Jesus.

§

Following is some of what I have personally seen, heard, experienced, and absorbed like a sponge from the folks I have encountered.

A thirty-five year-old mother of three is on maintenance. She is skin and bones, bald and frail to the eye. She has beautiful white teeth, a quiet demeanor, a wonderful smile, and a testimony that will win over the hardest heart.

She suffers through the harsh treatment just to stay alive another month or year to be with her family. She loves Jesus; she said so. She told me that her smallest little girl said to her one day when she was very under the weather, "Mommy, you're not sick, you just have cancer."

An older Catholic lady who prayed the rosary during every treatment befriended me and we prayed together and shared stories. She had a huge smile and spoke of her Lord and Mother Mary, and was so sweet, and gentle, and made me feel as though I was one important soul. I fell in love with that lady.

She has a story worthy to be a part of this book, and we have included it a bit later. We think you will be as impressed with her journey as we have been.

A twenty-two year old, beautiful lady, wrapped in a blanket, to whom I gave one of Lynn's books, told me how her boyfriend broke up with her when he heard of her cancer.

She looked into my eyes and asked a piercing question. "Who would ever want me?" I almost broke down at that point, but I was able to recover.

I told her Jesus wanted and loved her and I cared about her also. I assured her there was someone out there with the right priorities that would want her for who she is, not what she is. She smiled and hugged me. I fell in love with her too.

Being a retired Navy Senior Chief Petty Officer, I always notice military people in uniform. I noticed a very nice looking young man walking out of the infusion room. He was in the uniform of a Navy Lieutenant. We talked Navy stuff and I said goodbye thinking he was there with someone.

I saw him again a month later. He was wearing Bermuda shorts and I could see he was missing a leg. He had come for treatment. He smiled and came up to me and we chatted for a few minutes. He was a pilot, I saw his wings. I don't know the rest of the story, but he had a great spirit.

An African American lady, maybe in her nineties, was being infused and appeared to be just one step away from heaven. I looked at her and smiled, and she shared with me her life-long struggle with cancer that had invaded every part of her body. But she loved Jesus and bravely faced every day as a blessing. She was weak and sick, but she had an inner strength that set her apart from many of the other patients I have interviewed.

An older African American gentleman smiled at everyone in the infusion room and said "God bless you." As he departed before I did, I noticed he could barely walk, seemingly from a bad leg. He spoke to others as he left, nodding his head in the affirmative and waving.

A very thin older lady was shivering in the chair next to me. I asked her if she had a blanket, and she replied that it was her first visit and she didn't realize it would be so cold.

I found a WINGS volunteer and she brought a blanket for the lady who smiled at me and mouthed the words "Thank you." I was beginning to catch the wave of serving my fellow cancer survivors.

I'll stop here with the stories and say that I forgot my own woes while I was ministering to others. In fact, I felt pretty good.

Judy and I went to the grocery store that week and bought a ton of snacks and brought them in for the WINGS volunteers to hand out.

I began to live outside of myself and projected what I had into the lives of others. Some would die and find their healing in heaven.

Some would live on but never be what they once were. Others would never be totally free of cancer, and many would see it return again and again. That changes one's focus to the present and away from the future.

§

I am no stranger to pain and suffering. Besides being a cancer survivor, I had a near fatal motorcycle accident some ten years ago in which I suffered fourteen broken bones, a broken back in two places, a collapsed lung, tendon damage, and a concussion. That put me in the hospital for three weeks. Healing time was about a year, and there was a great deal of pain involved.

I have had thirty-six broken bones –all legitimate accidents. One doctor asked me if I had fallen out of an airplane after looking at my history.

I've been electrocuted nearly to death when I tried to do some electrical work while standing on an aluminum ladder. My arm turned black where the electricity flowed through my hand and out my elbow.

As a child, I contracted a near fatal fever from a community swimming pool. Had my head nearly removed when a boy on the school playground swung a ball bat that connected with my face, breaking my jaw at the age of nine. My jaw had to be wired back together.

As surprising as it may seem, I was plagued with a facial tic for thirty years. Hemifacial spasm is a neuromuscular disorder characterized by frequent involuntary contractions or spasms of the muscles on one side.

These were embarrassing to say the least, and the treatment ranged from painful Botox injections to an inhumane test called Electromyography or EMG. It is a technique for evaluating and recording the electrical activity produced by skeletal muscles.

EMG is performed using an instrument called an electromyograph, to produce a record called an electromyogram. An electromyograph detects the electrical potential generated by muscle when cells are electrically or neurologically activated.

The signals are analyzed to detect medical abnormalities, activation level, or recruitment order or to analyze the biomechanics movement. This is a long way of saying they stuck large needles in my face in different places and then shocked me about eight times –trust Jesus.

That's enough of my medical history for now. I say all that to indicate that I understand protocols, pain, terror, and disappointment. None of the treatments worked for the facial tic. I lived with it long enough to learn to live with it.

Then I began to pray about it, and God did not answer my prayer the way I wanted Him to. Instead, he brought to my memory the Bible verse in 2 Corinthians 12:7-10 about Paul, who had a thorn in the flesh given to him to keep him humble. Three times he prayed for the thorn to be removed. God said no.

That was not really what I wanted to hear, but I accepted it and went on with my life. One day, maybe fifteen years ago, I got up and went through the day without a tic. Next day was a repeat of the day before, and the next and the next until today. God took it away in His own time, but not until after I resigned to having it and would still function as a teacher, etc.

§

All healing or lack thereof is from God. Life is filled with injuries, diseases, deformations, bodily function disorders, and system failures –life goes on regardless.

We can have joyful productive lives as we learn to compensate for shortcomings, faulty functions, handicaps, and limitations. It used to bother me when people would stare at my tic, and I knew what was going through their mind. After a while, I said to myself and God, *"If Paul could do it, I can do it."*

In fact, people with handicaps or physical limitations are known to develop exceptionally advanced skills that outshine "normal" people –whatever that means.

§

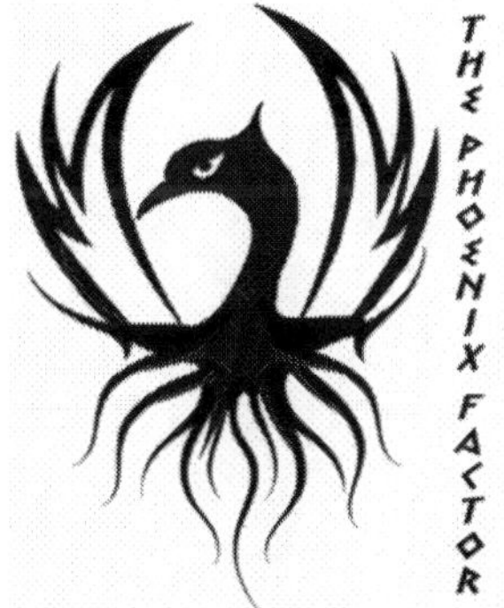

Learning to be thankful for what we have and not focused on what we do not have, or have lost, is vital to a satisfied mind and happy heart.

It can only be learned through practice and reestablishing priorities as God gives grace for our personal situation. Grace is unmerited favor,

Godly strength, and wisdom to live life to the fullest regardless of circumstances.

§

Scripture Verse. NIV, God said in *2 Corinthians 12:10. "But he said to me, 'My grace is sufficient for you, for my power is made perfect in weakness.' Therefore I will boast all the more gladly about my weaknesses, so that Christ's power may rest on me."*

§§§

Chapter Eleven

This Little Light of Mine

The nights were sometimes pretty bad, but often times the days were worse. Darkness seems to synchronize with woes and despair, and depression. So do rain and winter weather. They don't battle each other, but act in harmony to allow the blues to come, the tears to fall, and the angst to spice up the lot.

As I lay motionless in the recliner, even my thoughts were dull and lifeless. My prayers seemed often to be exercises in futility, and my only real pleasure was watching the travel channel, cooking shows, and the show that presents the star eating unbelievably bizarre foods. But they helped pass the time –lots of time.

As the last treatment began to subside and mellow, I could do some things in a limited way. A wheel chair borrowed from our church gave me some mobility, because I was too weak to walk. Our friend, Sheila loaned us a walker that I learned to use and for which I became thankful.

Against my doctor's advice, I went to church several times and even taught Sunday School –and picked up a couple of bad viral bugs that put me down hard.

My blood count was low, platelet's were low, and my immune system was totally south of the border. But it felt good being out and about. But they do tell you to stay away from crowds of people for a reason. They were right.

It was sort of humorous in a way as I sat in the back of the church during the service. After it was over, the folks would come by and want to shake hands, which I refused in a polite way.

Some would throw out a passage of Scripture and run; some would smile and wave; some would just stare, not knowing what to do.

I was invited to a fish fry at church hosted by another Sunday School department. We went and sat at a table as the fried fish, fried hushpuppies, and French fries were served. I tried one very small bite and had to leave. Oh well, at least we went.

I began to feel pretty much worthless and pointless. I had been gobbled up by the 125 billion dollar a year chemo therapy industry and I was just another patient with a number.

I would wait and wait, sleep, take my meds, wait some more, pray for bowel movements, try not to fall as I walked to the bathroom, and nearly gag as Judy brought me more water to drink, and drink, and drink.

One day, Judy and I decided we would read Lynn Eib's book, When God & Cancer Meet, aloud together. We read and talked and read. Lynn's story, individual survivor stories, Scriptures, helps, encouragements, and even those precious souls that died made for things with which we could identify.

Lynn spoke to me and to Judy in the lines of her book. She had been there and she knew the ropes. She shared, she explained, she guided, she understood. *I love you Lynn Eib.*

As I licked my wounds and as Judy tried to overcome the shock, fatigue, frustration, and confusion of our state, we both began to see the flicker of a little light in the dark distance.

Our desperate prayers had been answered; our friends had come through many times, prayer support from all over the United States continued day and night, things changed for the better, even the protocol iterations changed to be more considerate and supportive of our needs.

We learned that pain, trauma, agony, dissipation, invasion of false modesty, interruptions in schedules, plans, and future vision didn't kill us, but in fact made us more patient, accepting, and strong.

I dropped my guard against intimacy on a whole different level, in which the most delicate life concepts, functions, and relationships were discussed more openly and honestly.

We stripped away much of the fluff that normally accompanies conversations, and got to the point quicker, more considerately, and openly, making what people could do for us easier, more available and even more to the point.

Things did begin to change after a while. In fact, I changed more in a little less than a year, than I had in my whole lifetime. Some things about us just won't change unless some factors change first.

Someone said of the prisoners of war of times past, that they all developed a philosophy of *don't sweat the small stuff, and it's all small stuff.*

I guess that when guards are waiting to beat you for the least provocation, there is no toilet paper, no open communication, no food or water, and one doesn't know from one day to the next if you will live or die, nothing else matters much.

To the POWs, family was way out there somewhere. Home was even farther away. And sitting in the rain became a sensual pleasure as you bathed in it, become purified, cooled, and rejuvenated by the falling water. The rest was all small stuff.

I gave up on longing for food after about ten days. I learned to appreciate the nutrition drinks, and my beloved even toiled with foods until she lucked up on something I could swallow and keep down –like slightly sugared oatmeal.

Minutes of surreal daydreaming and passing of time turned to hours, to days, to weeks, and then to months. Life hung on and pleasures came from the strangest places.

Neighbors came to visit and one friend cut our grass and raked our leaves for the entire season –free-gratis.

Another neighbor trimmed our bushes and one kept our front yard clean. Many were the times old friends and new ones came by for deep theological discussions, prayer, and light hearted conversation that produced laughs.

Our youngest granddaughter brought her favorite stuffed animal for me to cuddle with. She created hand made cards, and my oldest granddaughter posted uplifting messages about me. I was made to feel important and loved –but from a distance, so to speak.

I am an avid lover of New Orleans and Louisiana based mysteries by one particular author. As I read his work, I can experience Louisiana from my recliner.

I can smell and taste the seafood, feel the rain and winds, hear the local dialect being spoken by the characters, smell the oyster shells piled in the streets, see the shrimp boats in the bay, hear the Zydeco music from the shanties, and watch the dancing and carousing that has made the French Quarter famous. I can taste the café au lait, beignets, and strong Cajun coffee.

As badly as I needed diversion, I even stopped reading my favorite fiction author. Cancer and chemo can strip you of just about everything, and leave you with just about nothing if you allow it. I did at times succumb to the ravages, but I overcame them much of the time.

But the cards, calls, e-mails, visits, electronic social media messages and posts kept coming, and kept me going. Judy kept my meds coming on-time, made sure I drank my nutrition drinks, and kept the water flowing –trust Jesus.

And thus was the life of Michael Eugene LaRiviere, cancer survivor, and Judith Diane Wilson-LaRiviere, cancer survivor and care giver.

As time passed, so did many of the terrible things that had filled our days. We both learned that we could do without a lot of things we previously thought were necessities. We reprioritized what was really important.

We became appreciative of others and each other. We did what we didn't think possible. We began to be thankful in the midst of cancer.

I began to see people differently. I began to notice facial expressions, the looks in their eyes, the concern on their face, their desire to do something for us, but what?

We began to listen to what people were trying to say versus what they said. We gleaned a great deal from their intentions. We accepted their best efforts like apples of gold. We became very thankful for our friends, even the ones we had never met.

This is going to sound like I am bragging, but people began telling us what blessings we were to them, and how they appreciated our testimony and giving God all the glory.

It made us feel special and quite good. We were making a contribution to others, even in our weakened condition. We began to feel a developing purpose for our situation –perhaps even a calling.

We began hearing of friends who had contracted cancer and were frustrated, fearful, and all those other emotions I have listed so far in this book.

We would send cards, call them, talk with them, give them one of Lynn's books, pray with them, and offer to be there for them. Things were changing and so were we. All the things that seemed so negative to Judy and me turned out to be opportunities to develop resilience and endurance.

It has been my experience that people, including me are afraid of suffering and will take extreme measures to keep from suffering at all –but we are not promised a suffering free life.

Suffering has helped both of us to become more human and humane. It allowed me to focus daily on God's goodness, grace mercy, compassion, love and power.

Suffering has prompted me become more tolerant and helpful of and to others and has allowed others to become more tolerant and helpful toward Judy and me. As I end out this chapter, I want to leave you with a few thoughts that are most important to grasp when it comes to finding the purpose for suffering among the saints of God.

God teaches us that through suffering we are meant to go deeper in our relationship with Christ. We get to know him more fully and deeply when we share his pain.

As a writer and Bible teacher, I create and share most deeply and sweetly about the preciousness of Christ when I do so through what I have endured for and with Him.

§

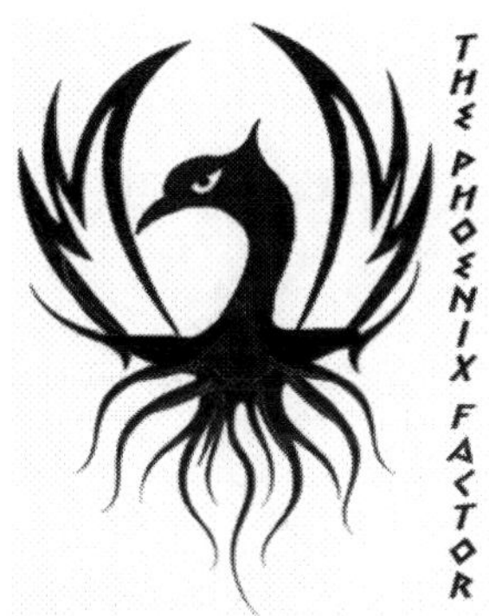

Before cancer, my priorities were different. When I am now called upon to choose between the world and Christ, I choose Christ. If I lose any or all the things this world can offer, I will not lose my joy or my treasure or my life, because Christ is all I have and want and to do His will is my highest aspiration.

§

Scripture Verse. *Philippians 3:7-10. [7] But whatever were gains to me I now consider loss for the sake of Christ. [8] What is more, I consider everything a loss because of the surpassing worth of knowing Christ Jesus my Lord, for whose sake I have lost all things. I consider them garbage, that I may gain Christ [9] and be found in him, not having a righteousness of my own that comes from the law, but that which is through faith in Christ—the righteousness that comes from God on the basis of faith. [10] I want to know Christ—yes, to know the power of his resurrection and participation in his sufferings, becoming like him in his death, [11] and so, somehow, attaining to the resurrection from the dead.*

§§§

Chapter Twelve

Saying Goodbye is Painful

Cancer, treatment, and all the trappings in a strange sort of way become old friends, and one becomes used to them being around. We live with and through them; our schedules always consider them, and our very being finds a dependency in them.

Then one day the sun comes up on a brand new day, and it is different than the rest. Almost imperceptibly, God has announced a significant change in what has been a lifestyle.

The phone doesn't bring as many calls from friends that center on cancer or care giving. Cards, meals, visits, and social media references to our situation are all drastically reduced.

The change settles in after a few hours and when bed time comes, it is with mixed emotions that obviate something missing or that it is incomplete.

As the days pass, I realize that I'm not the center of attention as much any more, as morbid sounding as that might be, and Judy isn't giving status reports to neighbors or our social media friends.

Bushes remain untrimmed, chores remain undone, and visits diminish. It's almost like the world around us has breathed a sigh of relief as its attention is drawn elsewhere.

§

Concern over world issues, war, starvation, the plight of Middle Eastern Christians, Israel, local news, rioting, the border crisis all begin to creep back into our daily life as significant issues that merit our attention and concern.

I begin to notice that we need a new mattress because where I slept has begun to sag. I have just about worn out my beloved's recliner, the carpet is in need of replacement, and the house seems to be crying out for new life.

The atmosphere of somberness and the aura of melancholia seem to be lifting, and colors begin differentiating the highlights of our home.

We go back to church to a receptive family greeting, and I get my head rubbed with its new batch of hair providing a scruffy bristling feeling. Folks smile, tell me how great I look, and I suddenly gain an affinity with pregnant ladies whose tummy seems to be public domain for pats and rubs.

By now I am actually seeing people as they greet me, and I am actually hearing them as they speak to me. I even remember what they say.

Now I'm hearing more and more from others about what a miracle and inspiration I am and have been, and how God brought me out of the deep crevice that cancer had thrown me into.

We returned the wheel chair to the church and the walker to Sheila. The cancer related supplies that a friend whose husband died of cancer had provided were returned.

We donated my extra trach supplies to the Home Health organization for use by folks without insurance. And the last trappings of emergency catch pans, paper towels for mouth wiping, cough drops, and plastic water bottles have been removed.

One thing I noticed was that I wasn't watching the Travel Channel and the cooking shows anymore. That is one psychological phenomenon that I will think about for a long time –how a starving man can enjoy watching food preparation.

I started eating oatmeal, cereal, soup, noodles, some cheese, and toast. My taste had not yet fully returned, but my revulsion for food had seemingly disappeared.

My bowel activity had not returned to normal, but I no longer experienced impaction or ten days between reliefs. I could shower without passing out, and I was getting hair back all over my body.

I worked up to getting up and down the stairs to my home office, around and about the yard, and we had started reading books aloud again and studying about things that interested us – like heaven, a closer walk with Jesus, and opportunities to serve others.

Judy could return to her Bible study at a nearby church, go out on her own; have lunch with friends and gain a bit of pleasure in some private time, without worrying about my well-being.

§

Things were returning to *normal* again, but I realized that I no longer knew what *normal* was. I didn't worry about insignificant issues like I used to. Jesus had an open line to me, and Judy and I prayed together more often. The Holy Spirit filled our home and we liked it.

Frustration, fear, anxiety, and disappointment seemed to dissipate and resignation to whatever remained allowed us peace of mind.

One thing I think you might find interesting at this point is that at the start of my journey, Jesus told me (in my mind) that I would not die, but I would suffer a great deal for His glory and honor.

I had forgotten that a couple of times, when I thought I would die, and was looking forward to doing so. I remember what He said to me now, and I had to chuckle in a way when I thought back to the reality of His message to me.

I can't pull the cancer card out anymore to get sympathy, get out of work, or be the most significant person in a room. I look fairly normal, eat pretty much what I want, and am back to living a regular life on a normal schedule. Let me elaborate on something I just said.

Eating has become interesting. When I got my taste back, I couldn't get enough of my favorite foods. I never felt full. Normally, people begin to feel full after eating a meal –not me.

I have gained back fifteen pounds and have to make myself stop eating. Especially sweets like pies, cakes, cookies, iced anything, pancakes with loads of butter and syrup. I went from one extreme to another –from starvation to gluttony. So I have to watch the diet.

§

As I grew in strength and clearness of mind, Judy and I felt more and more that we were being called into something special. We attended a monthly cancer support group at West Clinic under the shepherding of Reverend Sharon Herlihy.

This monthly get-together involved watching an excellent video about going through cancer and treatment; we prayed for each other; we told our stories, ate great snacks, and fellowshipped.

One other fellow and I sing, and we have a spirit-filled worship circle of black, yellow, and white –we are still missing red. Numerous denominations, prayer styles, temperaments, sensitivity, and experiences all mix to produce an amazingly wonderful time of encouragement, hope, vision, and shared testimonies, failures, fears, joys, and personal victories.

Men and women in attendance pray, weep, laugh, remain silent, and drink in the overflow of strength that fills the room. Sharon brings an exceptionally mature leadership and control to the gathering.

Sharon adds spiritual insights, Scripture reading, intercessory prayer, and guidance. When we finish, very few run out –they want to stay. I have a saying that "people do what they want, do what they believe, and if they like something, they will be there."

I think that the greatest draw for Judy and me was the freedom and enthusiasm of worship style and expression that each person seems to feel. We are awed at the way they glorify

God and reflect His care and love for them through cancer, suffering, experience, and victory. You really have to be there to fully understand what I am trying to convey in words.

Judy and I believe that the responsibility of every born again Christian, regardless of denomination, is to reflect the love of God in Christ to the world, so that people will want a relationship with Him. It is not as important to quote Scripture as it is to reflect that Scripture in one's life so that others may see it fleshed out.

Folks around us have a need to see Jesus reflected in the lives of people who are experiencing pain, loss, discomfort, insecurity, and who do not know just what their future holds.

Very sick folks may not know exactly what their future holds, but their attitude toward life does reflect their confidence that God holds their future and guides their path in the present.

§

Judy and I have begun discussing our experience with newly diagnosed patients and care givers. We will be working in a cancer support environment in the future, and have done a great deal of introspection designed to help others make it through what we have already experienced.

We asked ourselves and each other what it was that we needed most when we were going through the wrath of chemotherapy. Here's what we came up with.

- Recognition as to our significance
- Appreciation as human beings
- Support in doing the things we couldn't do
- Encouragement, positive insights and thoughts

- Communications: e-mail, cards, calls, social media
- Concern: expressed, implied, obviated
- Prayers: individual, collective, verbal, electronic
- Offers of help and willingness to follow through
- Acceptance even with our issues
- Solid friendship: visits, chores, transportation, food

One thing I learned from the experience is that no matter how badly I may be hurting, how weak I may be, how sick or frustrated I am; that is no excuse for abusing or forgetting the needs of others.

I don't have to thoughtlessly act out my own discomfort and project it onto others. Life does go on, and as yucky as I may feel, I still have to live it and realize that there are people who are watching me and need me to be strong, objective, and as pleasing as I can be –like our granddaughters.

It sounds like a huge responsibility, but I may be the only cancer sufferer that someone sees or with whom they have a close association as they begin their journey. I may leave them with a sour taste in their mouth, a defeated attitude from the start, and a hopelessness that someone else will have to undo.

One great truth I can share here is that I am so thankful that I was able to make it through this experience, not having destroyed any relationships in the process.

I can look people in the eye and thank them for their service to my wife and me. I can smile at friends and not have to be ashamed of my conduct with them. I can shake hands with well wishers and know they were not offended by my attitude.

You may think those things are trite or trivial, but once angry, hurtful, bitter or thoughtless words are spoken, they cannot be taken back. They are out there and have already caused damage and perhaps destruction of relationships. Even though we may apologize, those words are still lurking beneath the surface waiting to rise unexpectedly in a future crisis.

§

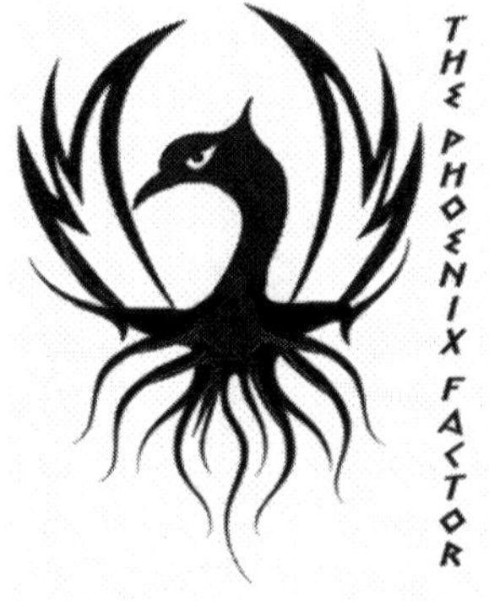

There are a lot of thanking and expressions of gratitude that are due, cards to be sent, calls to be made, and kind words to be expressed to friends, neighbors, family, relatives, and folks we have never even met. It means a lot more to be able to do those expressions of love and thanks when the heart and conscience are clean.

Scripture Verse. *1 Thessalonians 5:18. Give thanks in all circumstances; for this is God's will for you in Christ Jesus.*

§§§

Chapter Thirteen

This is My Story – Sylvia Schulker

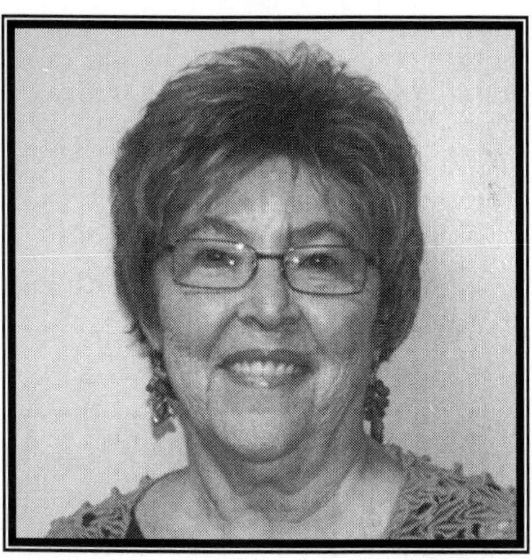

Mike. A few cancer survivors have crossed our path that have something different in their lives; something that sets them apart from others. They have a spirit of light in the journey that takes them through the dark night of the soul.

We've known Sylvia for many years, and she has always had a strong faith, character, and testimony. We asked her to tell of her experience from the perspective of before, during, and after her fight with cancer. This is her amazing and encouraging story.

If I were to bundle what she told us into a hymn of praise, I would use two lines from an old song, *Blessed Assurance* by Frances J. Crosby, written in 1873.

This is my story, this is my song
Praising my Savior all the day long

§

Silvia. My husband Ed, who happened to be a minister and I always placed our service to God at the center of our lives. Sometimes though, like many other folks, we would stray and seek directions or paths that were not necessarily God's personal choice for us.

Somehow, the Lord always got our attention, and like the Good Shepherd He is, drew us back into the flock. I look back now and realize how much I depended upon Ed in the leadership role of the Godly man he was.

On March 2, 2009, Ed was admitted to the hospital with a diagnosis of pneumonia. We weren't overly concerned as he had been sick for over a year; with no alarming diagnosis.

That night was different –he was placed on a ventilator and put into an induced coma. The doctors said his body needed this to help regain his strength, because he had suffered a heart attack.

Later they told me he had acute lymphoblastic leukemia, lung cancer and congestive heart failure. Now I knew why he had been suffering so for the past year. I never got to say good-bye to my beloved, for he never woke up. I was angry and bitter; why did no one know?

I began the dark, dark path of grieving for the one with whom I had shared fifty-three years of marriage and had known since we were seven years old. My husband, my best friend, my partner, was gone from my presence.

The sudden loss of Ed took me to the depths of suffering, pain, loneliness and darkness. I wanted to pray, but couldn't. There was a wall between God and me –one I had built in my grief. It was like a fire had ravished my life, and I was left sitting in the ashes.

I would go to church, but just a hymn that he had loved would bring sobbing tears and I would have to leave. That was a time in my life that I really needed God; but for some reason, I couldn't reach up to Him.

Gradually I began to read in Psalms and pray the Scriptures, but still a dark veil separated me from my Father. One verse in Psalm 30:5 became very special to me. *weeping may stay for the night, but rejoicing comes in the morning.*

After almost a year, I realized hope can rise from the ashes. I would get through this time of grief and become a wiser, stronger and more effective servant for our Lord. Little did I know what I was facing in order to become that person.

§

Cancer – The word that changes a life –either in drawing the survivor closer to God or causing the victim to become bitter. It is the word no one thinks he or she will ever hear; but it often develops and comes to us under a veil of darkness. Sometimes quickly and then sometimes it seems to lie dormant, erupting like a volcano. That is the way cancer entered my life.

Sunday morning, February 14, 2010, I started to get out of bed and get ready for church. When my feet hit the floor I had this terrible pain in my right side. Thinking I had pulled a muscle, I waited until Tuesday, the 16th, before seeing a doctor. He became extremely concerned and sent me directly to the hospital.

After many tests, I was scheduled for surgery on Friday, as they had found a large mass in my colon. I asked the surgeon if he thought it might be cancer and his reply was, "We are 99% sure it is."

§

Even though I was hearing words I never thought would be spoken to me, God took over and gave me a peace I cannot begin to explain, or even understand, for it was the *Philippians 4:7. peace that passes our understanding*. I truly had no fear as I was taken to surgery.

After several hours in surgery I was taken back to my room where my daughter, Tracy, was waiting. The doctor came in and told us the cancerous mass was as large as a man's fist. The cancer had gone through the colon wall to the appendix, small intestine and the ileum. It was also in the lymph nodes.

He explained the surgery required removal of a large portion of the colon, the appendix, and small intestine, plus several lymph nodes. Still, God's presence is filling that room with His comfort and peace. He never left me.

My daughter later told me, "Mom, I thought you would really fall apart, but you accepted it in a way I couldn't believe. When you showed your faith, then it made my faith stronger to deal with you having cancer."

She had seen my grief—depression—tears—over the past year and didn't think I could survive the news of having cancer. But, she saw how God was working through this.

It seemed as though my walk with God changed drastically with the diagnosis of cancer. I began to pray *Philippians 4:6-7.*
6 Do not be anxious about anything, but in every situation, by prayer and petition, with thanksgiving, present your requests to

God. [7] And the peace of God, which transcends all understanding, will guard your hearts and your minds in Christ Jesus.

I again felt the presence of Almighty God in my life. My focus changed from the darkness of grief to the need for my Savior. The reality of my life being completely in His hands became real again. He was everything I needed.

The Word God gave me that day was *Isaiah 41:10. So do not fear, for I am with you; do not be dismayed, for I am your God. I will strengthen you and help you; I will uphold you with my righteous right hand.* How I praise Him for all He was doing as I walked through that deep and dark valley.

§

After recovering from the surgery at home, I sought God's will in choosing an oncologist for the chemo treatments I was facing.

The clinic I thought was the best never returned my phone calls. Yes, God was working! I found the name of a doctor that a nurse had written down. I called and they saw me the next day.

Psalm 138:8. The Lord will fulfill His purpose for me... He did. I know God led me to this oncologist for I had that special peace as we discussed the treatments and tests. He explained he was going to be very aggressive in my treatments.

I would face six months of chemo –some really rough days, but each day I learned to trust more and more as God and I walked through this time. I praise Him, even now, for the many blessings He placed in my life through other patients being a blessing to me and allowing me to show His love to others.

I wanted to be a testimony of what God means when we trust Him for our every need, and believe me; cancer will bring a person to this trust. I only wanted God to be glorified in every aspect of my *walk with cancer*.

One of the most difficult issues through this time was not having my husband by my side. I can't really explain in words the loneliness I felt at times. But, God knew, and He began to fill the emptiness in my life, and truly became my everything.

Zephaniah 3:17 says, *The Lord your God is with you, the Mighty Warrior who saves. He will take great delight in you; in His love, He will no longer rebuke you but will rejoice over you with singing.* It still amazes me how God spoke to me through His Word every day.

On my visit in November 2014 to the oncologist I asked him if I was in remission, or what my status was right then. He said, "Sylvia, I consider you cured!"

Cured is the "C" word every cancer patient wants to hear. I told him it was all God and how God used him. He expressed to me for the first time, the surprise my recovery was to him. He didn't think I would be able to walk into his office without a walker, after the six months of chemo.

That night as I wrote in my diary, I praised God for all He was and is to me. He brought me out of that deep valley of dealing with the big "C" and now we were on the mountain top.

Hallelujah! My verse to Him was *Psalm 77:14. You are the God Who performs miracles; You display Your power among the peoples.* Amen and Amen. I don't know what the future holds for me; but I do know Who holds my future.

§

God worked many miracles in my life and I just wish I could explain in words just how much He means to me today. Through the cancer I began a very personal relationship with my Father.

A few years before my husband died I had to have serious eye surgery. The surgeon told me if I didn't have it that week, he probably couldn't seal the hole in the macular.

God had led me to this doctor in His time and yes, He was in control of the surgery. I was on the brink of going blind, but He touched me in a special way. I tell you this as it plays a large role in why I didn't think I could ever be of service to God.

After the cancer, I began to have terrible back and leg pain. I was diagnosed with a ruptured disk. Many weeks of pain, hospitalizations, tests; and yes, God again performed another miracle. No surgery; just nerve blocks, and I am now pain-free. My daughter said she was beginning to think I was another Job.

Even though I was faithful in attending church services, I never thought I would ever be able to be used in service. My body was still weak from the chemo treatments; my eyesight was not as good as it was before the surgery, but God can take the weakest vessel and use us.

I often thought of Paul and his thorn in the flesh that never held him back. Moses with his speech problems and God already had Aaron prepared to serve. My prayer was, "God, if you can take this piece of clay and mold it into something useful to your service, then I am willing."

He did the best He could with this weak body and now I am teaching a lovely group of ladies in Bible Study on Sunday mornings. You see, I had given up –that was me. God never gives up on us. I have to pray every day for God's strength; both physically and spiritually, for His wisdom and guidance in my walk with Him.

He has blessed me beyond words and I praise Him for the awesome God He is and for all He can be to anyone if only they trust Him. I had to learn to let go and let God. Being a Christian is not getting what we want. It is recognizing God's authority to give us what He knows is best.

At this point in my life, I can honestly thank God for my cancer. It changed my life completely in regards to my relationship with our Father.

I learned what it means to give everything to Him in complete trust and faith. My daughter, Tracy still tells me over and over how my faith gave her strength in dealing with me having cancer. She felt she had just lost her daddy and when the diagnosis came about stage three colon cancer she thought I would fall apart.

Tracy didn't realize that I had already turned it over to God and had peace like I had never before experienced. I always took strength in my husband Ed's preaching and teaching and his complete yielding to God. He was such an example in his faith.

Why I can say, "Thank You God for cancer." God revealed Himself to me in so many ways during the year I walked this horrible path.

One thing I am sure God knew troubled me about my husband and his leukemia. It was one of the first things God revealed to me. If no cancer, then I would never have made my peace with this question. I often thought Ed could have been treated had the doctors diagnosed him correctly. But, here God was working and I am so thankful.

The first day I took my chemo treatment, I sat in a chair next to a lady named Sylvia. We began to talk and she said she had leukemia and had been treated for five years. Her words to me were, "If I had known what I was facing these five years, I would never have started my chemo."

I looked at her frail body—almost down to just bones and oh, so weak. I realized God had planned this moment just for me. I began to visualize my husband in this situation and I knew that God was telling me through Sylvia that Ed was removed from that kind of suffering. In this, I thank God for cancer.

I thank God for cancer as it brought me out of the despair of grieving –drawing into myself. I was now restored to *the joy of His salvation.* I have a testimony of the awesome God we serve for He is more real to me today than ever. He is my constant companion. I kept a diary and each day I wrote how God had blessed me. This I wrote on October 18th:

> *Father, God, I consider this whole cancer deal worth it, if in the end I look and sound more like Jesus. Some days are pretty ok and some are really tough, but it's all worth it if somehow I can honor You in going through this experience. Whatever the outcome, please be glorified.*

I experienced His love in ways that I had never known before this year. He truly clothed me in His blanket of peace—the peace that Paul tells us is available to all if we just pray. I prayed over and over the special comforting verses of *Philippians 4:6-7.*

Also, my faith became stronger for I had to trust God for everything. Walking by faith means being prepared to trust where we are not permitted to see. People who did not know the Lord were placed in my path on this journey and I was able to share what God was doing in my life.

When you have cancer some think it is like a dark cloud hovering over you; but God allowed me to look beyond the clouds and see His glorious working in my life.

Without cancer I would not have the intimate relationship I now share with our Lord today. I am changed! When I first began to pray over the cancer I was praying for a miracle---that was me. But, when I gave myself to Him; He took control and blessed me far beyond the miracle of healing.

§

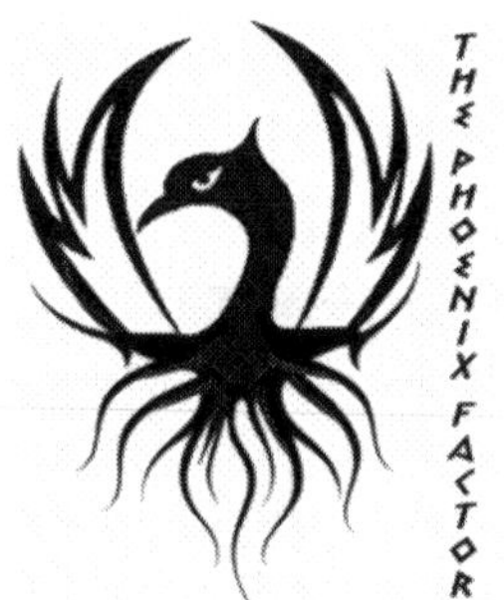

I wasn't prepared to take the journey with cancer without Ed, but God gave me wisdom, strength, and assurance, and I still praise Him and thank Him. Oh what an awesome God we serve!

§

Scripture Verse. *Psalm 116:1. I love the LORD, for He heard my voice; He heard my cry for mercy. Because He turned His ear to me, I will call on Him as long as I live.*

§§§

Chapter Fourteen

Mutual Support - Rick and Sharon Perry

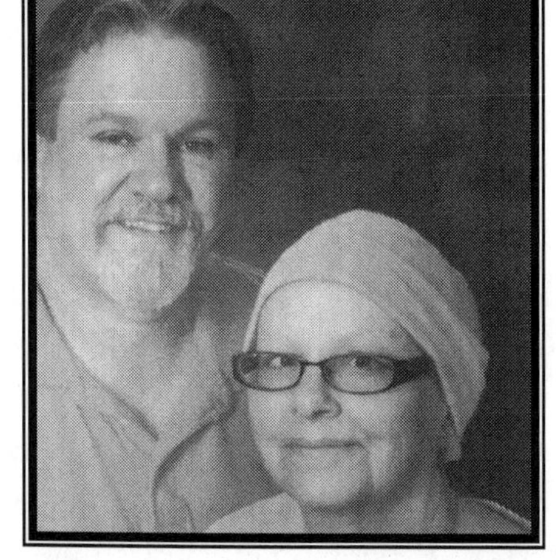

Cancer is a hard journey on a rough and dark road.

It's frightening and frustrating, physically and emotionally dissipating, and takes the cancer patient to the ends of his or her patience. What used to be is no longer, and what will be is unknown.

Cancer and its treatment, as brutal as they may be, are also spiritually maturing, life changing, and reprioritizing of those things that are really important.

Ours is a story of what it means to be a cancer survivor and a cancer care-giver. It's an attempt to tell of emotions, love, support, and learning to give up what we can't control to God; to trust Jesus; to acknowledge God's sovereignty, and to become comfortable with our own human limitations.

§

Sharon. My name is Sharon Ann Perry, and I'm a fifty-three year old mother of three grown children. My husband is Rick Perry, the fifty-three year old father of my three kids, the loyal and untiring lover of his wife, and the unrelenting protector and provider for our family. That's really how I feel about my beloved.

On November 20th, 2013 I was diagnosed with breast cancer at the Church Health Center in Memphis, Tennessee. That day marked the time when my life grayed out and I was hit over the head with a load of bricks. My past disappeared, my future became a big question mark, and everything focused on the present, and all that could be summed up in one word; cancer.

During a routine self-examination, I discovered a large, hard lump in my left breast and immediately went to a trusted family friend and physician, Doctor John Albritton, who set our wheels in motion toward what I am today –cancer free.

When reality had a chance to set in, the first thought that I can remember rushing through my mind was *will I die?* It seems funny to me now, but I started receiving numerous life and burial insurance advertisements in the mail to which I had previously paid no attention, but now stimulated thoughts of whether or not I needed it, and *how did they know?*

The protocols set up by the team of physicians that would care for me were temporarily delayed because I contracted the flu; was put on antibiotics, and could not begin the treatment process for another week –it was waiting time—that was such a long week.

I'll never forget how God was quickly and prominently injected into my journey in such a way as to bring Rick and I comfort in our time of distress.

A female surgeon that we called Doctor Z was educating us on what to expect, and when she had finished, Rick asked her if we could pray. Doctor Z dropped to her knees, as did we, and we prayed right there. That launched the next phase of our journey with new confidence.

§

Both Rick and I would often find ourselves thinking about The Footprints Prayer, an inspirational poem about having faith in God. Also known as Footprints in the Sand, it shows how God is always with us, especially in times of need. But it really helped to build our confidence to watch and hear a doctor pray for us. That became for us one of the first footprints in our journey along the sandy beach called cancer.

Rick's father died of prostate cancer in 2009, and for the last three months of his dad's life, Rick acted as a care-giver for him. Rick has often mentioned how strong his dad was during the entire ordeal, and how it had taught him that he couldn't fix everything, and that tears were okay.

I won't go deeply into the treatment of my cancer; the side effects of chemotherapy have already been explored in the front of this book. Suffice it to say, that the author and I suffered many of the same issues, and experienced many of the same emotions.

I had eight chemotherapy treatments totally including four *Red Devil* shots of a thick chemotherapy that we affectionately renamed the *Blood of Jesus*.

§

The chemo worked to rid me of the tumor, but a mastectomy was ordered and performed, and now I am healing, regaining my hair and strength, and am rejoining the normal world. But the story doesn't end there.

Not long ago, I worked up the courage to look at myself naked in the bathroom mirror after a shower. What I observed was that I was totally hairless and missing my left breast, which left me with a large gouge where my breast once was.

It's very hard to describe my feelings. I still have not allowed my husband to touch the area of my surgery. It's hard enough for me to touch it. As I viewed my image in the mirror, I felt incomplete. A woman's pride is enhanced by her hair and breasts. I had lost both. A bit of shame shot through my soul as a bolt of electricity and chill ran through my bones.

I remember wondering, *who am I? I have to protect my family from my mastectomy.* I just wanted to cover up the gouge with the gauze bandage and not look at it.

§

Before cancer, both Rick and I were normal, average Christians who went to church, attended Sunday School, prayed, and performed many things ritualistically, but with only minimal fire and fervor. We were content and felt secure in knowing we would go to heaven when we died. That would all change.

I was in charge of the house; I cooked, washed, cleaned, and did it all while my husband made a living. That would also change. Today, we do everything together. My husband is my best friend, my main support, my love, my prince.

My mom and dad are deceased, our kids have moved away, and we have the empty nest. I must say that when our children came home as their lives permitted, my spirits were lifted, my strength renewed, and my heart warmed. They may live away from us in distance, but they remain very much a part of us.

We have another family that came through for us during this trying ordeal that was there for us, that supplied our needs and supported us –our church family. Each member who contributed anything to us helped to make the transition from then till now possible.

During the cancer diagnosis, treatment and follow up stages, I noticed things had changed in our lives. I had gone from a five centimeter tumor, stage three breast cancer, to being cancer-free but missing a breast and temporarily my hair.

On a positive and somewhat whimsical note, Rick says I have the smoothest skin he could remember since we had been married –chemotherapy and loss of hair do that. I guess maybe it's a kind of payback for taking so much away. I didn't even need to shave my legs, and that was a plus.

§

What have we learned in all this? This is where cancer divides patients into those that become victims or victors, survivors or sucumbers, bitter or better people. It robs or gives a Christian witness and testimony.

For us, we have learned that God is in control and is sovereign. We trust Jesus exclusively, and rely on Him for everything. We feel so much closer to God and feel His presence every day. And we have both learned to be still and listen to Him.

§

I will say that the one of the most frustrating or frightening things centered on the installation of my portacath. I remember being transported down a long hallway and through swinging doors into a room filled with silver and white things.

Before I could pray, the oxygen mask was placed on my face and the anesthesia took over. When I awoke, it was over. I learned afterwards that my Sunday School teacher was praying for me the whole time I was in surgery. That was one of the things that bolstered my spirits.

The highlight or highpoint of my journey came when the doctor told me I was cancer-free. I could now heal and recover knowing the dreadful thing that had threatened my life and body was gone.

My church family has become most important to me, and I remember once speaking with Mike and Judy LaRiviere, and coming away feeling a little better knowing that I was not alone in this ordeal; that others had lived through it. That's the way it has been for us. *No-one can fix me, but they can sure help me.*

I don't want to sound critical in any way, but this comes from my heart. I don't get very much out of well-meaning folks who spout Scripture to me. I really would rather know what that Scripture has done for them and how it can apply to me.

Scripture can be empty when used because someone has nothing else meaningful to say. Sometimes silence is best, your presence is most meaningful, your words are not always necessary. Just be there.

I think that for me one of the really saddening things centered on the times when I felt like a leper with a bell around my neck. I would watch as people I knew would look out of the corner of their eyes and see me and go the other way. I know they were having trouble dealing with my cancer and surgery. I knew, but I was still hurt by it.

In retrospect, I think that perhaps information could have been a little more forthcoming about getting prostheses wigs, special bras, and an artificial breast used until I have reconstruction surgery. This type help is up to the people who provide support services to cancer patients. How well they do their jobs is up to them.

In closing this part of our story, I have learned to look at Rick and realize that even he can't fix me, he can't control the outcome, and he can't work miracles –but Jesus can. What Rick could do is remain strong in the Lord and fight the good fight with Jesus as his *Psalm 91:4. Shield and Buckler* –and he has done that to perfection.

§

Rick. I have changed for the better through all of this. I was a professional wrestler at one time, and I learned all the tricks to fighting bigger, stronger, and more ferocious opponents in the ring, and winning.

Cancer proved to be the biggest, strongest, most ferocious opponent I had ever faced, and I simply could not win against it. It countered my every move; it overpowered me, blocked my best maneuvers, and seemed to know my plan and thwarted it.

Cancer pinned me very fast, but just before I was counted out, Jesus stepped in and took over the fight. But I did walk away with bruises and bumps.

I have learned patience; how to relinquish responsibility; that prayer does change things; how to find blessing in each day; and how to be thankful in all things.

I watched my sweetheart open over three hundred cards and sometimes wipe a tear, smile, and even just stare at what was written. As long as we have been married, I still can't tell just what goes on in my bride's mind. But I can tell by looking at her when something tugs at her heart strings.

Cards came from all over the country, as did calls, e-mails, social media posts, and visits. Food was overflowing, friendship flowed freely, and encouragement came from everywhere. There is a lot of goodness in this world, and a lot of wonderful people.

We have grown so much spiritually; have learned to turn things over to God and let Him keep them; but most of all I realized that I don't love Sharon for her breasts or her hair, I love her.

I'm not so naïve as to think a man can understand the loss of a breast, but at least I'm okay with it. I also learned to periodically find a quiet place to cry and let the tears wash my emotions –it does feel better. I do remember how great I felt just for a moment, as I came to the full realization that *God's got it!*

I think the low point for me came after the third chemo treatment when I asked Sharon why she wasn't dressed and ready to go for her next treatment.

She told me she wasn't going; that she was through –finished. I didn't know what to do, I felt so weak and inadequate. She finally changed her mind, and we went. It did show me how tough it had been on her, and how tough she really is.

§

In ending my part of our story, I just want to say that after experiencing what we have gone through and what we have become, I would never want to go back to what we were before cancer. God has used this to grow me up and grow us closer together. *Thank You God, for Cancer!*

It's always encouraging when you find out that your dark journey toward the light has helped someone along the way. We were both so blessed when we received a social media post from a friend. She gave us permission to use it in our story. Here it is in its entirety.

> *Mrs. Perry,*
>
> *Hi, this is Amy Trim.*
>
> *To begin this post; I received a package today from a woman I've never actually met, for my baby that is on the way. Technically, we are family through marriage, but we've never even spoken on the phone. Since hearing of my pregnancy and our struggles, she's become one of my biggest advocates.*
>
> *The amazing part of this to me is that this person is and has been going through her own personal struggles. I just couldn't imagine her going through them and also taking the time to care about someone else who she's never actually met. This woman's strength is beyond amazing to me, and her caring heart goes beyond words.*

In like manner, I can not put into words how appreciative I am for all the things you have done for my little family. It is amazing that someone I've never met has gone out of her way to be so kind. Actually, it's refreshing and is something I wish everyone got to experience so they could also believe in humanity again.

You're an amazing person, and I know that about you through my association with your daughter. A lot of times children are a reflection of their parents, and you have an amazing daughter.

My husband wants me you thank you from him as well. Our relationship has had a lot of obstacles but with God and people like you in the world I think we'll all be just fine.

Again, thank you and God bless you and Mr. Perry.

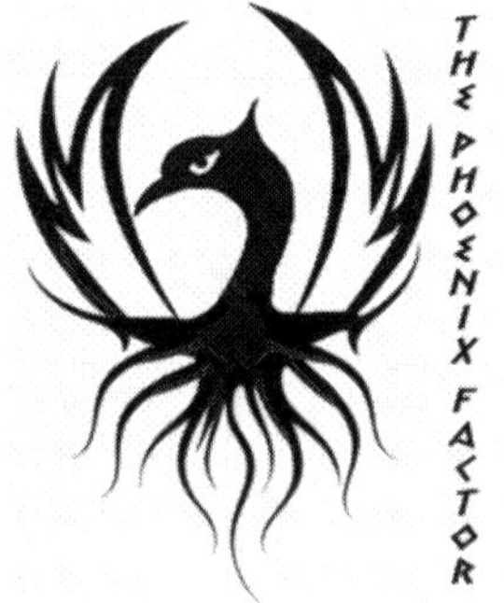

It was a tremendous blessing for Judy and I to visit with Sharon and Rick in the hospital when Sharon underwent reconstruction surgery.

This was the beginning of another leg in their journey as she heals and looks forward to a future free of cancer.

§§§

Chapter Fifteen

Journaling - Joyce and Rodney Dayley

Mike. I took an interest in Joyce Dayley as I read her social media posts, and became drawn into her sweet but powerful spirit and acceptance of the journey on which God has placed her.

Her journaling of the end of life experiences for her and her beloved husband, Rodney are too precious not to be shared with a broader readership.

I reviewed her website at: www.youravon.com/rjoycedayley and found that she had interwoven her life and business in a unique way that had led to her being quite successful as an independent Avon Sales Representative. In fact, she is among the top twenty-four sellers within the Avon community. It prompted me to look deeper.

It is my sincere and heartfelt pleasure to be a part of bringing to cancer survivors and care givers, this treasure of victory, blessings, faith and hope. Thank you, Joyce, for your willingness to have your story told.

Joyce speaks of blessings many times, and how she and her husband, Rod always look for them on their journey. She, Rodney, and their family are among my greatest blessings.

Rodney Dayley was a *blessed* man to have Joyce Dayley as a wife and caregiver. There are many similarities in the Dayley family journey to that of the LaRiviere family journey. I am a blessed man to have Judy as my wife and caregiver. God has not yet called me home, but when that time comes, I hope that I have as much peace as did Rodney. God bless you both.

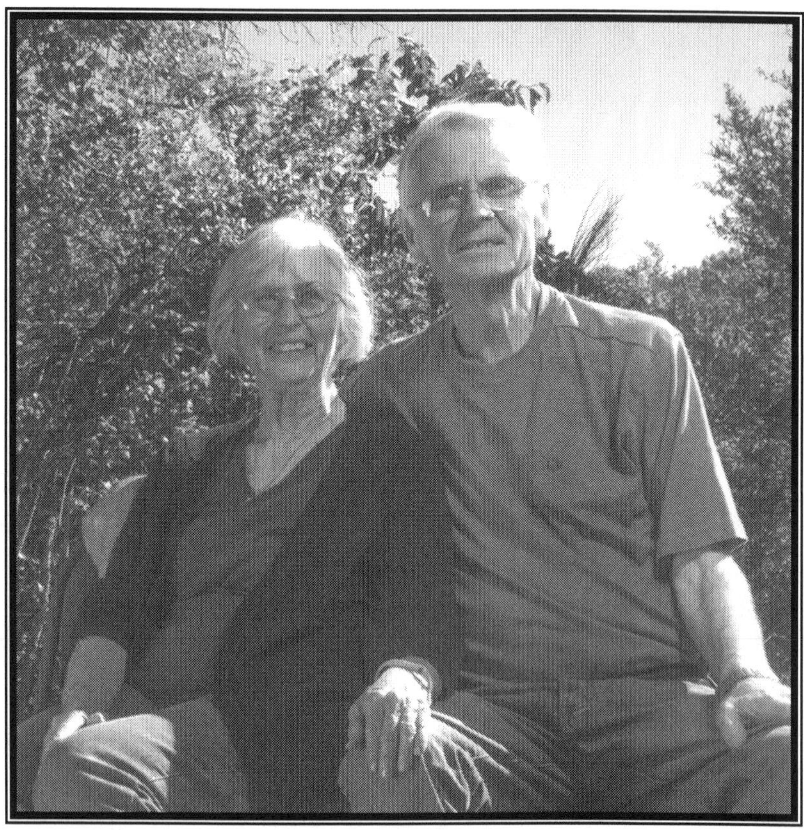

Joyce. I have a confession to make before we get too far into this chapter. I've been a writer since my teens, but it was only during this journey that I have shared my writings with more than a handful of people.

A friend of mine said that she had been touched, and that her life had been changed because of my journal. I have had people contact me concerning what these stories have meant in their personal life, and when Mike expressed his desire to share it in this book, I was deeply touched.

Today makes four weeks that Rod has been gone, and I find myself looking up into the heavens more often than ever before. My therapy is writing. I write to him almost every night before I go to bed. I just like to keep him up-to-date on what is going on in this earthly life.

Some of my writings are too private to share on social media, although at some point I do intend to return to writing on a more regular basis on my private page of Good, Better or Best.

I have shared with some of my friends about having this chapter in Thank You God, for Cancer; they all ask when it is expected to be out.

In my communications with Mike and Judy, the authors of this book, I have come to the conclusion that writing a book must be a lot of work –writing about my feelings for therapy reasons sounds easier.

§

I am sixty-eight years old, and have a special needs daughter that I adopted when she was four and a half years old. Her name is Diani. She was born normal, but was abused as a baby which led to brain damage. When I adopted her, I was told she would never intellectually pass the two year-old level. She functions now at about seven to eight year-old level and is the love of my life.

One day I will write a book about Diani and the many lessons I have learned from her. So I am not completely alone now. When Rod used to take overnight business trips, I slept with lights on and had great trouble sleeping. Now that he is gone, I do not leave the lights on, I also sleep like a baby. I think it's because Rod taught me during the last few months of his earthly life to learn to be comfortable with the quiet. Besides, Diani keeps me company.

Rod taught me that the Spirit teaches and comforts during the quiet times, and my home is filled with so many memories and love that it has not felt empty at all. My biggest fears were the night, quiet and emptiness, so overcoming those has been a blessing beyond measure.

Our cancer story began in 2003 when I first contracted breast cancer. That was the year I thought my life was ending, but in reality that was when it really began. I lost my hair to chemo and lost a breast, but I found courage and hope, and learned I could do really hard things with a lot of support, prayer, and faith in God.

My Husband said, "Honey, it's just another adventure and we are doing it together." He was amazing and he supported me in doing the Avon Breast Cancer Two Day Walk in New York City in 2004 and 2005. We left our comfort zone, and did what we had never done before.

In 2014, we were asked to step out of our comfort zone once again as Rodney was diagnosed with pancreatic cancer. Therefore a new cancer adventure had begun and ended ninety-three days later as my beloved husband graduated from the school of very hard knocks, and went to his reward in Heaven.

The following is the journal I shared over social media for a little over three months. It literally allowed me to vent and to deal with my emotions.

Day 1 - April 28, 2014. This morning I woke up at three thirty and could not get back to sleep. I have been trying to post on social media, but my computer keeps shutting down. My husband is having a test done at the hospital this morning.

I have a slight headache. So I think it's time to turn my day around and go on a scavenger hunt. I know there are many things to be thankful for, and I am going to see how many I can find. I will take my pen and paper around with me all day so I can jot down all the things I find to be thankful for. May we each be blessed to find at least one thing to be thankful for today.

Day 2 - April 29, 2014. We learned yesterday that the Computerized Tomography or CT scan for my husband Rodney indicated that he indeed has pancreatic cancer and that it has spread. We are firm believers in miracles and prayers, and even though this does not sound good, we have seen and had many miracles in our lives and know there will be many more. We seek great inner peace and calm as we travel this road.

Yesterday on the way to Rod's CT scan, I told him I was looking for blessings, so if he saw any to let me know. He pointed to me and said "There's one," and then he mentioned how beautiful the mountains are. We counted many blessings on the way to the hospital and I knew I had married the greatest blessing of my life.

I truly have the most perfect husband ever for me. When we married in the Atlanta Temple almost thirty years ago, it was not until death do us part, but for time and all eternity. We agreed that we did not have to agree on everything, but we did not have to fight about what we did not agree on. That has made all the difference in our marriage. He is my very best friend who always treats me like his very best friend.

The CT scan did not pinpoint the ulcer we suspected and were looking for but did disclose pancreatic cancer that has metastasized into his lymph nodes.

By late afternoon he was thinking something was not right with his leg. His foot started hurting Sunday morning, and we decided we needed to go to urgent care because he had knots on his leg.

They sent us to the emergency room and there he was assigned an angel of a doctor who sent him for more tests that discovered two blood clots in his leg. He also went many extra miles and found us a cancer doctor and set up the appointment for today for us (another blessing) He treated the blood clots and told us what needed to be done. Our two boys, Gabe and Terry and our daughter Traci were there helping take care of everything.

The report we got does not look good, but with that being said, we have great faith. It is our prayer and hope that this will be another way for Heavenly Father to show the world another miracle, but he and I both know without a doubt that we have a Heavenly Father who loves us with all of His heart and He will always be there for us and with us.

We are sad, but we have inner peace and calm amid the storm we are experiencing. We are looking for the beautiful rainbow that appears after the storms in life.

When I went through breast cancer eleven years ago, we shed some tears, actually more than a few, but Rod said "We are on an adventure and we will find the treasures along the way together." And we did.

Day 3 - April 30, 2014. Wow, here we go entering into day three of a new life for the Dayley Family. It seems that the last two days were about two months long. We have shared tears with many of you in person or on-line as we have heard hard things from the doctors.

We thank you all for taking this journey with us. We have shared our thoughts and feelings and have been amazed as the prayers have rolled in from so many places. They came from my third grade school teacher; to grade school friends I have not seen in fifty to sixty years.

Each post and prayer has lifted us, as I have shared each one with Rod. The Lord often uses journeys like this to show us how precious life, family and friends are in our life.

We human beings are not mind readers and that's why it's so important to share our good and hard times in the most positive way we can. That allows us to come out of our world of being so busy and see the reality of pain and joy around us and then that allows us to step outside of ourselves and serve.

Just so you know prayers for another person in pain is service. I have read each and every post to Rod as you post it and with each one he has smiled a smile of love and thankfulness for your love.

A biopsy will be done tomorrow, Thursday morning, and after a few days we will know more of our plan of action and I will share that with you. I am thankful to know tears are alright, because right now we have had many and seen many and we love you for your tears and prayers.

Day 4 - May 1, 2014. Getting ready to go to the hospital for Rod's biopsy, and my friend Becky had shared this on her page. I just had to borrow it to share also. *I am so thankful for the gift of life that Heavenly Father gives to us each day. My Mom who died at age ninety-one used to say, "First thing in the morning I check the obit page in the newspaper and if my name is not there I knew it was going to be a good day."*

The Dayley's are going to have a good day today. And if you are reading this, you are going to have a good one also. Embrace the day and share your love.

Day 5 - May 2, 2014. How can day-five seem like it has been months long? Yesterday was Rod's biopsy and the people at the Provo Hospital could not have been kinder or nicer to us while we were there.

As the shock factor starts to fade and reality starts to set in, it is a lot like living with a tornado and you just try to stay out of the path of negative thoughts and fear and hold close to the Savior as you prepare for the storm.

Our faith in the Lord is our storm shelter we have been given in which to seek protection as the storm passes –we are safe in the arms of our Lord. Negative thoughts are like opening the doors of the storm shelter and allowing the storm to come into a place that is safe and secure.

So as we hold fast to what we believe we still have fear, we still shed tears but we know we are not left alone and we have a safe place to be.

Rod and I have read and reread the many comments you have posted; we have felt your prayers and love and it has made us stronger. We are not strong, we are not brave, we are just normal everyday people who have been asked to travel a road we would rather not be on but if we have to be on it we are so thankful for so many dear and kind people are willing to take this journey with us and just know that we are lifted by your love.

Day 6 - May 3, 2014. Rod, I and three of our kids, Terry, Gabe and Traci, met with our doctor yesterday afternoon and we listened to the results and the road map he laid out for us.

It is pancreatic cancer that has metastasized. Surgery is not an option –so treatment is basically chemo or nothing. Either way the time afforded him is four to twelve months.

Doctors only know so much. A few years ago they told us to come see my Sister Mary Ann "now" because she had a week at most. They did not know my sister. She was with us two months. God is still in charge –not us and not the doctor.

Tears pop in and out. Just as do weak and strong moments. We are on an emotional roller coaster; but to be honest, most of life is just that. So we will ride the ride and be so thankful for the overall peace that our faith and knowledge in our Savior gives us in our heart.

We will have many more tears and we will have many happy days filled with laughter and making more memories that we will cherish forever. But today the Lord has given us a happy day.

Our daughter Diani turned forty and we are having a birthday party tonight to celebrate her turning *old.*

She is so excited and so full of fun and laughter and happiness. We will completely bask in this joy with her as we celebrate her Birthday.

She is a gift the Lord gave us thirty-six years ago and she continues to bless our home each and every day. So today, cancer goes on the back burner as we celebrate life and living and make some wonderful memories.

We don't know just what decision we will make for Rod's journey. With so many people praying and fasting for us tomorrow, we know it will be the right decision for this family and this journey. Thank You to our church, Cedar Hollow Second Ward, for holding a special Fasting and Prayer for the Dayley family's comfort and healing.

Day 7 – May 4, 2014. My amazing husband's journey continues. Yesterday was very tiring for him as it was Diani's fortieth birthday party and even though it made him very tired, he loved seeing our angel having so much fun.

Thanks to our Home Teacher, Brother Packer and his Wife Connie. You kept Diani going with so much laughter. She loves you both so much. We were so blessed to have so many friends come and share in this celebration and some of these friends we had not seen for years.

Today with much Fasting and Prayer being offered up for Rod and our family, we know the spirit of the Lord will be stronger than ever and we want each of you to know how much we love you.

As we fight against this storm in our life, we are learning how to sail our ship and how to stay closer to the calmer waters of believing in our Heavenly Fathers plan. He is in charge and loved us so much He died for us so that we can live again. The storm may be raging but when we stay close to the Lord, it truly calms the waters of doubt and fear.

Day 8 - May 5, 2014. Yesterday was Fast and Testimony Sunday with many of our friends all over the world fasting and praying for Rod and for our family to have comfort and healing if possible. May I just tell you we felt every prayer, we felt your love and we felt your good and tender hearts?

Today is a new beginning, and we shall take a deep breath and start again to search for the blessings the Lord has prepared for us just for today. I have no doubt they will be there and we will find them.

Day 9 - May 6, 2014. What a wonderful blessing to have a family home evening with our children and grandchildren and to feel the love and strength that comes with song and prayer and a lesson.

We are so blessed to know that families can be together forever. We are so happy to know we don't have to be perfect to be happy. Time spent with family is like heaven on earth.

Rod and I married in the Atlanta Temple for time and all eternity and we had each other plus six children between the ages of eight and fifteen full time. What a roller coaster ride we have enjoyed for almost thirty years. And the icing on the cake is fifteen grandchildren that are our greatest blessings. Thank You God for such a wonderful life.

Day 10 - May 7, 2014. Still praying for miracles; that is how we live our life, and seeing new miracles each and every day is what we do. We have always believed that you do not always get what you asked for but we have always gotten just what we needed. And for that we are so thankful.

Yesterday was such a wonderful day. It was an almost a normal day, and that was a blessing. Sometimes we forget that normal can be so wonderful. So we will take each and every normal day we can get. We thank God for today and every gift He has given us; the gift of a normal day of life filled with love and laughter and joy.

Day 11 - May 8, 2014. Have you ever lived in the *tomorrow I will* way of life? I think we all do. Do you ever save the really good china dishes to use someday when it's a really special day? Do you tell your family members how much you love them every day? I am realizing more and more that is a normal way for most of us to live.

Diani often says "Mom, you are so busy". That should be a clue that maybe it's time to slow down and smell the roses. When life throws you a curve you were not expecting, it looks a little different and you start to think a little differently. Your bucket list starts to look different also. The things that really matter start to come to the surface.

We are slowing down and coming to an understanding that today is a really special day. Today would be the day to use the really good china; if we still had it. We got rid of it years ago, since we hardly ever used it. Now we are saying *today I will* instead of *tomorrow I will.* We share our thoughts of the memories we have made over the years and relive them.

Through our sorrow, the Lord gives us better vision to see that the really important day is today. Perhaps, if there is something you have really been wanting to do, make time to do it now.

Today is the day we see the oncologist and get the full report of Rod's biopsy and make some decisions for our *today and tomorrows*, so a few extra strong prayers will be helpful today. Thanks so much for your prayers and well wishes.

Day 12 - May 9, 2014. Yesterday as our sat in our doctor's office, we wondered what decision Rod would make as the doctor told us that without chemo his time would be short; weeks to maybe six months; with chemo maybe nine to twelve months.

The doctor said the chemo he thought would be best for this was a low dose chemo with manageable side effects; once a week for three weeks; off a week and then three more weeks and off a week and then another scan. If the treatment was helping we would continue if not we would stop.

We felt this was acceptable since we want him with us as long as possible. Since I have been the chemo route eleven years ago, I am not a fan of the treatment. I was amazed at the peace that filled my heart with that decision. I knew that whatever decision Rod would make would be the right one and we would have no regrets.

Today we go to the hospital and have a port put in, which will make the chemo much easier for him and next Thursday we begin his first treatment.

You often hear the term *dying with cancer*. We have decided we don't like that phrase so we will be *living with cancer*. We will make each day count by living fully with the peace of our Savior, we will also live with humor and laughter and thankfulness for our many blessings and putting as much life in each day as possible.

I will continue the post of his updates as much as possible for those of you who want to read them. Please remember I do them mostly for my own therapy.

Day 13 - May 10, 2014. I am so thankful for a Mom and Dad who taught their children to have faith in the Lord. During our life time we have to have faith and knowledge of who is in charge. We have to have faith that His love is so strong that He will carry us through whatever is placed before us. Yesterday our son Terry took us to the hospital for Rod to have a port installed.

Rod did very well in the morning, but as the day went on he became extremely tired and a little confused. The afternoon brought more blessings as help came from friends and family.

We are weak in so many ways, but the Lord has given us strength that we never knew we had. For that we are grateful. As I continue to share your posts with Rod. He smiles when he thinks of each of you and how you have touched our lives.

Day 14 - May 11, 2014. I used to think normal days were boring and very uneventful –I was so wrong. Yesterday was close to a normal day filled with normal thoughts, feelings and actions. Thank you, God.

Last night I had one tired but happy husband who had worked in the garden all day and had a somewhat normal day. It was wonderful to have a good day with Rod. I am learning that a normal day is a gift from God.

Day 15 - May 12, 2014. It is a difficult day for Rod with a lot of pain. Much of the day was spent in bed sleeping and freezing. By night time he was warm and the pain had eased and we made it over to the kids for part of the Mother's Day celebration. The grandkids entertained with music: piano and singing and lots of wonderful drama put into their singing.

Can I just tell you what a blessing it is to have children and grandchildren for a girl like me who grew up wanting to be a wife and mother? When I told my dad that I wanted ten kids, he said, *Why would you want to bring kids in this world when there are so many already here that do not have homes?*

So Dad planted the seed of adoption in my mind. It made sense to me. So I knew I would not only have children, I would also adopt.

I began the adoption process from Korea where I found my little girl first, Sook Hee Lee who I renamed Traci Lee. She was twenty-two months-old. I thought she should have an older brother and that was when I found Goh Young Kim, who was renamed Terry Dean. He was three and a half years-old and had his shoes on the wrong feet.

Little did I know I would never have children of my own, a few years later we added Diani to our home while living in Oceanside, California. Nine years of marriage ended in a heartbreaking divorce and two years later I met and married Rod Dayley in Memphis, Tennessee. He had three children, Shelley, McKay and Gabe. Thus I had become a mom to six and grandmother to fifteen and had never given birth.

Day 16 - May 13, 2014. Yesterday was another almost normal day with a nap in the middle of the afternoon. Rod still had pain but he spent a little time in the garden which he loves so much. He also spent a little time at work just taking care of some loose ends. I drove him because he cannot drive due to the pain meds.

The thing that was not normal was a visit to a funeral home to get information on the cost and planning of a funeral. But that too was not a bad experience, just not one we expected to have for many years.

I have learned over the years that prayer really does work and it really does give inner peace that we cannot get anywhere else. I had a dear friend message me asking the secret of how we get through each day as she has her own private battles.

My answer was very simple. We turn our life over to the Lord, we pray and we look for blessings and look to see the hand of God in our life each and every day and thank Him. May you have a blessed day and see every blessing that the Lord has for you today.

Day 17 - May 14, 2014. My husband has given our children every example of what a marriage should be and how you should treat your wife. The only fight that they ever saw us have was staged as a teachable moment.

Six kids were fighting with one another and so we staged a silly fight in the presence of our children. Rod yelled at me, slammed the door and departed. I in turned, ran upstairs with my hands over my face. The kids thought it was to hide the tears; it was really to hide my smile. You could have heard a pin drop.

The kids were shaken and scared because they had not seen this out of us before. When Rod returned a few minutes later, he came in the door and I joined him as we entered the family room filled with very quiet kids and we took a bow.

We said, *How did that make you feel? It makes us really sad when you fight.*

Our kids were pretty good for a few weeks after that lesson – lessons seldom last forever, but our children never saw Rod treat me with disrespect because he never did.

To us, it is important to work every day on becoming a better husband, a better wife and a better child of God. It is not always easy but I can tell you that it makes life a heaven on earth when you live with kindness, love, laughter, hope and making each day an adventure; not only for others but for yourself also. Mean words or actions can never be taken back even when we say *I am sorry.* They are always in the back of the mind for instant replay.

Day 18 - May 15, 2014. I am learning more and more each day how much I have taken for granted each and every day. How I expect to get up every morning and I expect my family to be there with me and for me.

Yesterday was a hard day in many ways and has helped me to see more clearly what a gift life is for each one of us. Yesterday a good friend lost her Mom. We learned on the same day that Rod and her Mom had cancer. Her mom went to heaven yesterday. My heart breaks for her and her family, yet it also rejoices as they are so thankful for the love this mom brought to them each day. My dear friends, may you and your family be blessed with inner peace today and always.

We did uncomfortable things today like attending a chemo class. Rod begins his first treatment today. Chemo is something that I endured twelve years ago when I had breast cancer and must admit I have no fond memories of chemo. My prayers are that he endures it much better than I did. It was during chemo that I came to understand the true meaning of *crying unto the Lord.* So my heart breaks for him for having to go through it.

Another uncomfortable thing we did yesterday was that our son took us funeral home shopping. The people were most kind and helped explain the different plans for Rod, myself and Diani for the future. I must admit we did find a little humor in our shopping and there was some laughter involved.

I bet you are thinking. Wow, I should have skipped reading day eighteen of this journey, this is so depressing; but I hope you can see it as just a part of our trip home.

We are still excited to be together on our journey and thankful that we are learning to live with cancer and still see the hand of God in each day we are given. We are so very thankful to the many wonderful friends who have sent us cards of hope, who have done many acts of service for us, have brought us food and have shared phone calls and private messages of hope and your own stories of your journey's and many other things.

One of the sweetest blessings is our children, grandchildren, our brothers and sisters and their tenderness as they reach out with so much love and service to make our pathway easier. Church members who are there with support, neighbors, long distance friends and those who are just minutes away. The sweet little neighbor girl who comes over and knocks on our door and say's, "I just wanted to say hi and we sit on the door step and chat for a few minutes". Then she is off to brighten someone else's day.

These are the things that make our pathway bright and full of love and hope. So yesterday was difficult, but it also had its tender moments. Our life is full of peace and love. Who could ask for more?

Day 19 - May 16, 2014. First chemo treatment yesterday was endured well by Rod. He is tired but so far not sick. When we came home his hope was to spend a little time working in the garden which he did –perhaps a little too long because he was really tired last night, but happy.

What got us through the day is the same thing that gets us through every day, the love of our Heavenly Father, the help of family and friends and all the many prayers that we say and prayers from each of you and many others. The things that were once important are still important but many of them we have learned are not as important as we once thought they were. I have often wondered if I would do things differently if I was told I only have a certain amount of time to live. The answer for us is yes.

We are learning that many of the things (stuff) that we could not let go of because someday we might use it or need it is just not so important anymore. When the things you own take over your life you learn that you no longer own them, they own you. So as we are moving at a slower pace during this time we are looking at what is most important for us so we can make better choices.

We are so thankful for the wonderful life we have been given, we are so thankful for a kind and wonderful Heavenly Father and for family and friends!

Day 20 - May 17, 2014. Rod was up early with some pain and I asked him what he would like for me to share in my writing. He simply said he was feeling loved, so thank you everyone for bringing such feelings of love into the heart of my husband. He did pretty well yesterday morning but the afternoon and evening brought on the side effects of chemo. Hopefully they will go away soon since he has to do the chemo treatments for three weeks in a row. Thursdays will be his chemo days. He then gets a week off and then starts the next three weeks of treatment.

You all have filled us with love from your many kind acts of service and just a kind word or the many prayers that are being offered for Rod and our family. May you feel the love that the Dayley family has for you today and may you always know that you have made a difference in our life.

Day 21 - May 18, 2014. The ugly chemo and pain meds are taking us down a path we hoped to not have to walk. Nevertheless, we are not alone as your prayers and our Savior carry us through. Hard night and morning, but we have hope that this day will end with sunshine in our hearts. May God bless you this Sabbath day, and never forget to thank the one who gave us this day.

Day 22 - May 19, 2014. I'm amazed as the blessings continue. In February of this year we went to what is known as the happiest place on earth, Disney World. What a wonderful time we had but I have learned that the happiest place on earth can be anywhere as long as you are with family and friends.

Last night Rod was admitted to the hospital and we were surrounded by family our home teacher and his wife and our wonderful bishop. We shared laughter, silliness and tears. It appeared that last night the happiest place on earth was the hospital. May we each continue to see the hand of the Lord in our lives each and every day.

Day 23 - May 20, 2014. Yeah, we get to go home from the hospital in a few hours. Home Health care and a walker ordered in case it is needed. Our own bedroom and bed sound so good right now.

Day 24 - May 21, 2014. I love counting the days as I post. Each day gives me new hope and I cannot help but be thankful for starting the day at home, having had a good night sleep in my own bed.

It was great to come home from the hospital but by afternoon we had another scare when Rod experienced chills and couldn't get warm. Then he became very hot with a temp of 102.5 degrees Fahrenheit. We thought his condition would send us back to the emergency room, but the doctor was able to give us some ideas of what to do and within about an hour the fever broke and has not come back. What seemed not to be a good evening ended in a peaceful night.

Day 25 - May 22, 2014. Round two of chemo starts later today. Yesterday was better for Rod for most of the day. Those crazy nasty chemo and drug side effects are just not so nice sometimes. But he said there had some really good parts of the day also.

It's such a blessing to have had our silly spunky kids grow up to become warm and wonderful adult kids who are ever so protective of Mom and Dad. They help in every way to make things more comfortable for us. Mix that in with warm and wonderful friends and you get a pretty wonderful world.

Day 26 - May 23, 2014. Doctors' visit went well. Problems were addressed, some answers were found to make Rod more comfortable.

Even though Rod is often in pain, he is also at peace. He has had many friends and the people he has known over the years call him and I hear him say the same thing each time. *The gospel is true and that is all that really matters.* He loves Heavenly Father with all of his heart and that never changes.

Our son-in-law said that there were so many good things coming out of this cancer. We continue to pray for a miracle and we continue to see many each and every day. We have high hopes for the new meds to give Rod days of continued peace and the ability to spend some time in his garden which he loves so much.

Keeping journals of our bright and dark days and rereading them later really help us to see the miracles in our lives. Be a journal keeper. It will be a great roadmap for the future.

Day 27 - May 24, 2014. Yesterday was a regular appointment with Rod's doctor. It ended up with us going to the hospital for X-rays and more blood work. Results were okay.

Tonight I was thinking about cancer and chemo and the things I hated most about them when I went through them twelve years ago. I could give you a long list.

I remember feeling like I had a really bad flu mixed with food poisoning for a long time. It was scary when I heard someone cough or sneeze because I knew my body no longer could fight off germs the way it used to.

I remember listening to people laugh and talk as though the world had not really ended. *Did they not hear me crying on the inside and wondering why my world had stopped? How could the rest of the world keep going?*

I really did wonder those things for a while and then the Lord blessed me with eyes to see that other people were hurting also. Cancer is not the only thing that can stop your world.

Now I am watching many of those side effects in my husband, the love of my life; I hurt deep inside. But I know that Our Father in Heaven will be giving him the gift of wisdom and compassion that will change him forever and he will touch more lives in magical ways.

We hate what cancer does to our body, but we love what it does to the hearts of our children, family and friends. It opens our hearts to prayer and brings us all closer to the Lord.

As we went for a walk yesterday, one of Rod's friends was driving down the street and pulled his car over to the side. He jumped out and came over to embrace Rod with a hug.

He said "I pray every night for you, and I am going to start praying every morning also." This dear man brought tears to our eyes with his outpouring of love. Another friend said her young daughter came home from school the other day really excited because she saw Brother Dayley taking a walk, with a walker, but taking a walk. She was so excited to see that Heavenly Father was answering their family prayers.

I am not a fan of cancer or chemo but I am a huge fan of the side effect it gives to many of us. It brings us to our knees in prayer and closer to God.

Day 28 - May 25, 2014. Yesterday was such a blessing in so many ways. It was calm and peaceful. Still full of the nasty side effects of cancer and chemo but also filled with family love and help. I drove to the store for a few needed items and when I came home I found Rod in his garden pulling a few weeds. It was such a wonderful sight to see him doing a normal for him thing.

Sometimes we just want the bad stuff to be finished. Let's hurry up and win this race, and we fail to see all the beauty on the way to winning the race.

I learned a lesson in 1981, shortly after a painful divorce. The kids and I moved to Arkansas to be closer to my family. We rented a furnished apartment, we had no car, and it was a very humbling time in our lives.

We lived close to the mall and grocery stores so we walked to the store when we needed food. The race was so painful. I wanted to see the finish line and have this race behind me. One day as we were walking to the store, my eleven year-old Traci said with great excitement, *Mom, look at that beautiful butterfly!*

Just think; if we had a car we would not have seen it. This melted my heart and my self-pity and I knew it was time to see this part of our life as a journey filled with exciting things to see and do.

During this *poor* time of our lives, about two years, my children will tell you that this was the happiest two years of their lives. That two years was one of the most priceless gifts I have ever been given. Sometimes the race is more priceless than the finish line.

So for today, I will try to remember how important the journey is and continue to look for the many blessings that are given to us each and every day. I am learning to embrace the *gift of today* and the sweetness of family and friends and the never-ending love of a kind Father in Heaven who helps me to see the simple joys of life. May you have a blessed day of worship and a deeper love for family, friends, and God.

Day 29 - May 26, 2014. I love it when I wake up and hear the words *I feel better than I have in a while.* Now if we could just find the magic pill that lets that last all day long. My husband has so much pain from the cancer and chemo and from the side effects to the drugs that are supposed to make him feel better. I have pain in not knowing how to keep him feeling good. My heart hurts for his pain but it rejoices because he has great faith and trust in God.

I am not sure just how to handle life; but my theory is put it in the closet and worry about it tomorrow. That's no longer working for me. So, I am starting to do what my mother did long ago. I start working on the things that should be done now.

I remember her going through a million pictures and sorting them into piles for us kids and actually giving them to us. So yesterday, I started doing that very thing. It was so refreshing to see the memories over the years and start piles for all six kids.

I went through a whole shoebox of pictures. The problem is I have about ten to fifteen large boxes still to go through. I also found a box of writings that I had done over the years since 1968. So I would say it is time to figure out what to do and do it now – one day at a time.

What are the things you want to do someday? When will you start? Why do we always think we have forever? I took a trip home to visit my parents in 1988 and on my way back home I wrote this:

> *As we taxi down the runway once again, this time to go home. I think, just ten short days ago I was on this same run way coming into Memphis. I wonder if this is like birth and death. It seems like just yesterday that we came down that runway called birth and when it is time to return to our Father in heaven, it may seem much the same, as we enter that runway once again to enter into death. I knew my ten days would pass quickly and there would be much I would desire to do. Much I would want to see, and I tried to put as much into one day as possible, so I would not return home wishing I had done more.*
>
> *There were many times I practiced patience when I didn't want to, but knowing my time was limited with my family, it was easy to keep my mouth shut. It was so important to be nice and kind to my wonderful parents because I did not get to see them often. Life must be much like this; so very short and so much to see and do, but for some strange reason, we think we have forever to do all the nice things later.*

So therefore I often forget that I am just on a short trip, my life on earth, and will be returning soon to Heavenly Father. I hope on this trip of life that I can learn to have more patience, be more kind and put as much into one day as possible so that when I return home, I won't wish I had done more and never got around to it.

Day 30 - May 27, 2014. Yesterday gave us good and bad. The good was having a physical therapist come and show Rod a few exercises that helped with his back pain and by giving him a massage that helped him be pain free and sleep for several hours.

When he woke up he felt great and wanted to go to the store with me to get some food. It was a short ride, perhaps five minutes in the store, and it wiped him out for the rest of the day. The lesson learned was that we should have stayed at home so he could have felt good for longer.

Another good thing: we had more kids come over and do more work around the house and yard that needed to be done. So happy we have six kids, and I may be looking to adopt more. So if you are fun and a hard worker, watch out, you just may become a part of the Dayley family.

Day 31 - May 28, 2014. I am so thankful when a day ends up better than it started. I don't know about you but when things do not look so good my mind likes to go places that are dark and hopeless. That is when I have to talk to myself and remind myself that just because it's dark now; it does not have to stay that way.

There is light just waiting to peek through. Sometimes I have to turn on the light switch. Yesterday brought lots of pain throughout the day for Rod; even turning over in bed was painful. So it was mostly a stay in bed day quiet day.

It is very hard for any of us to have cheerful conversations when we have pain, but night time brought some light as he asked for some canned peaches that a dear friend brought over last week. Then a little before midnight he asked for more peaches. Who would have thought peaches could bring so much light and joy into such a dark day.

Many years ago I learned the secret of how to get rid of darkness in my life. I learned that if I only listened to or read things that were uplifting, it helped keep darkness out of my life. So that meant I had to invite the Savior who is the Light of truth and goodness into my life. I had to ask for help. I also found that writing letters to God often helped. There is something magical about putting your thoughts and feelings onto paper. My mind is a dangerous place when I only entertain dark and hopeless thoughts. I do not always do this perfectly but I certainly try to do it often enough to be able to see clearly.

Day 32 - May 29, 2014. Yesterday Our Son Terry took Rod for his blood work and I ran errands while they were gone. When I came back, I found Rod enjoying the yard and garden and telling Terry what needed to be done. Thank You God, for such a wonderful sight. I just had to share this with you.

He had more peaches yesterday, plus a very interesting meal. They say your taste changes with chemo –it does. He said for lunch he wanted just a few tablespoons of cottage cheese, a few table spoons of pork and beans and a couple of tablespoons of potato salad with a radish cut up in it and milk. I know, you're thinking wow, what a meal. I think I will have some of that today. Hey, he ate it and was happy.

Rod had only one small nap in the afternoon. His pain was more manageable and it was a great day at the Dayley home. Sometimes if we are wishing for better days ahead we find out that the boring days were really the better days we had been wishing for.

We are learning to live one day at a time and find blessings in each and every day and that there were some days that at the end of the day the best thing about that day, was it was over.

Today is chemo day again, then not another one until June 12. He gets a week off and some of his family will be here and he will go to the Temple with his brother Kevin on June fourth. That is so exciting. Please pray that Rod will feel well enough to go.

Day 33 - May 30, 2014. Yesterday was a great day which is a strange thing to say about a chemo day. It was filled with many blessings and only a short bout with intense pain later in the day. The doctor was very helpful. He listened to our concerns, made some changes and really seemed to care. Love it when they see you as a person instead of just a patient.

When we were in the chemo room, there was an awesome patient and his wife. They are younger than us and have two teenagers still at home. He is going through a tremendous battle with cancer stage four and would be having nine hours of chemo that day. They had a most upbeat attitude. We had good conversation and laughter. What a delightful couple. The chemo room was filled with love, laughter and life.

Later in the day, Rod and I just sat on our deck enjoying the afternoon. Yesterday afternoon we were not busy. We just enjoyed the day. A friend of Rod's stopped in last night to check on him; what a wonderful visit. What a wonderful day it was.

Now we move into today. As I said my morning prayers, I thanked Heavenly Father for another wonderful day in advance. I then quietly tried to get up and on with my day. It was just a little before five am, and I heard my husband say, "good morning, could you please get me a little cottage cheese with two peaches and a little salt and pepper?"

I then knew Heavenly Father really had another wonderful day in store for us. We visited and talked while he ate and talked about what great blessings we have. He then wanted to rest for a few more hours.

So as we move forward with the day. If you see us, be sure and look for the twinkle in our eye as we know it is going to be a wonderful day, and we will be looking to see if you have a twinkle in your eye also.

Day 34 - May 31, 2014. We sometimes get to walk on a paved road. But lately we are walking where the flowers grow. Yesterday was mostly a paved road but toward the afternoon we left the paved road so we could see more flowers.

The second day after chemo is not always kind to the body. But we got through it. A really good thing is we took a walk in the morning and he ate really well most of the day. We call that a successful day.

We also had really good friends and neighbors that did our yard work yesterday. With so many acts of kindness we feel humbled and blessed each and every day. Rod has gotten several cards in the mail and that always brings a smile to his face.

I must share an act of kindness that took place a few days ago. I went to our bank and made a deposit and one of the bankers who is a very kind young man was busy helping someone else but took the time to say hello. He knows what we are going through right now. So a new banker helped me and I left to come home.

Within a few minutes my phone rang and it was the kind young man who had been helping someone else. He said I had not seemed to be my usual cheerful self and he just wanted to call and make sure I was ok. To me that is a sign of real customer service and kindness. How often do we listen to the still small voice that tells you to do something kind and actually do it? And all of a sudden you have helped someone feel less alone with the burdens they carry.

If your road is not smooth today be sure and look for the flowers that will be planted along the path.

Day 35 - June 1, 2014. Today my sweetheart and I have been married for thirty years. I am so thankful for this man who drove from Memphis, Tennessee, where he was living, to Jonesboro, Arkansas, where I was living, on April 2nd, 1984 in the pouring down rain to pick me up and take me to a nearby bank parking lot, put a pillow in a puddle of water and proposed to me with a McDonald's ring as an engagement ring and asked me to be his wife for time and all eternity. I said yes. Our son Terry used the same pillow many years later when he asked His wife Lorie Jo to marry him.

So to my husband I just want to say, "Thank you for all the rainbows over the last thirty years. I am so grateful for being treated like a queen and for having him be my best cheerleader in whatever I wanted to do with my life. Thank you for taking me to the Temple and for loving me for time and all eternity. I love you, Rod Dayley."

Yesterday was a wonderful day filled with much goodness. Rod took a nap; had a wonderful visit from dear friends, and then I took him to the a special spa in Lehi where he got a Massage which really puts new life in him. The day was filled with visits and packed with goodness. This must be what Heaven is like.

By night time the pain returned but he was able to get a pretty good night sleep only to awake at four thirty this morning asking for Ritz crackers and milk. He felt pretty good this morning and is now napping until time to get up.

Day 36 - June 2, 2014. I live in a wonderful world and it gets better each and every day. Yesterday was one of those wonderful world days filled with the love of God, family, friends and wonderful lessons learned at church. I just cannot imagine a Sunday without church and learning more of an easier and more meaningful life.

Each week by Saturday my bucket in life is starting to feel a little empty and then on Sunday it is overflowing with what I learn and feel at church. I can remember when sometimes I would go home on Sunday and think, *that was kind of boring.* But then I would realize I was looking to be entertained, not taught by the Spirit. God's purpose is not to entertain us but to teach us how to live a good and kind life so we can live with a purpose each day of our life.

Yesterday was such a wonderful day and our thirtieth anniversary was filled with so much to be thankful for; anniversary wishes, Rod making it through most of the day without great pain. He was able to go to church, his brother Robbin made it in from Texas in time to go with us, our daughter Traci and her family brought dinner for our anniversary, some really good friends from New Jersey came by for a visit.

Our life and day was so full yesterday and each moment was filled with the way life should be lived. One of the greatest anniversary gifts ever for my husband was when our dear friend from church showed up with jars of peaches. Rod started the morning off at 5 a.m. with peaches once again.

Lessons Learned from yesterday: Enjoy life and the Gospel and what it brings into our life. Cherish friendships, stay close to your family, and live each day looking for the hand of the Lord in our lives. It is always there.

Count your blessings and name them one by one. And last but not least, be a blessing to someone else. Share your heart and you will bless and be blessed.

Day 37 - June 3, 2014. The cancer journey is scary in so many ways, but it is a journey we do not take alone. We have turned it over to the Lord and have put Him in the driver's seat, and we are just along for the ride. He is showing us scenery we would have never seen if we were driving. He shows us some of the back roads we would never have taken because we would have been in too much of a hurry to slow down and enjoy His world.

Some of the back roads are bumpy but filled with great beauty. As Rod was eating his peaches and cottage cheese this morning at four thirty, I asked him what he would like for me to write about today.

He said about the peace that comes from turning our life over to the Lord! What interesting conversations we have as we discuss funerals and shop for tombstones and life and death and songs for funerals, etc. We no longer cry as we discuss these things. It is like we are planning the trip of a lifetime and we want to make sure we get everything just right before time to leave. Fear begins to leave our hearts as we turn more and more of our life over to the One who is really in charge and just live each day we are given to the fullest.

Remember, we are just along for the ride and trying to see all the beauty He is showing to us. With that being said, we still live with hope in our hearts for the miracle. We still experience the hole in our heart at the thought of being apart, but we are at peace with God's plan and will accept it whether it is to be a miracle on this side of Heaven or on the other side. Inner peace brings great courage to live in the middle of a storm.

Day 38 - June 4, 2014. Today is a day where our hearts will be shared with many family members at the Temple. Family is here from Texas, Idaho, Wyoming, and Alaska and we will gather together for a very special day where many memories of the years will be shared as well as our love for God.

Please pray that Rod will have the strength to take in all of the goodness of family. Rod's afternoon was hard but the evening brought many family members together to visit and it was wonderful to watch brothers talk about the good old days.

Day 39 - June 5, 2014. Yesterday was so full of family and friends and the morning at the Temple with family and friends and the Lord blessed Rod with a smile on his face all day. I think we each experienced a little bit of heaven being able to feel so much love and great blessings throughout the day.

May we each enjoy a day filled with the people we love and keep a smile on our face as we move forward on the journey back to our Father in heaven.

Day 40 - June 6, 2014. We have learned that what we have been given is more than we ever needed and wonder why we never saw that before. We have learned that when the spirit tells us something is not quite right it is okay to speak up with love and turn a bad situation into something priceless.

When my sister, Mary Ann was on her cancer journey a few years ago, Hospice shared with us that even though cancer brings a lot of pain it also is a gift. Many people die quickly with no time for goodbyes, no time for the family to say what should have been said to bring peace to the soul. Cancer often gives us time to create many precious memories and remove any hurts that may have been stuck in our hearts over the years.

We have been blessed this week with some of the most spiritual lessons of our life. We have learned that our past has helped us to become who we are and that lessons learned over the years were stepping stones to bring us to where we are and who we are.

Day 41 - June 7, 2014. Beauty surrounds us each and every day and sometimes tears truly do come; not because we are sad but because we see goodness and beauty all around us. Beauty is in the sunrise and the sunset, it is in the clouds and in the rain, but most of all beauty is in our friends and family who share their love with everyone.

Sometimes the pain my husband endures is very hard but he works hard to manage it. He mentioned this morning how much he loves the beauty of the earth and all that is in it. God has created so much beauty for us to enjoy. Why is it so hard for us to see it?

We have watched television less over the last month, we have more quiet time sitting on our deck and seeing the beauty God has placed before us. A hummingbird warms the heart; taking a walk and encountering people that take the time to stop and say hello with a smile that brightens the sky.

We see neighbors with food in their hands going to see a friend that just came home from the hospital. A friend offers to take Diani to a program. Seeing service in action is beauty in action. May we each be blessed with eyes that see the gifts the Lord has ready for us today.

Day 42 - June 8, 2014. How often do we look at someone's problem and say, *There is no way I could handle that!* And then it becomes your problem and you learn that with God's help you can handle whatever you are given because you are never expected to carry it alone.

One of my daughters who was going to help me manage my busy day yesterday said, "Mom, it is really hard to be served isn't it?" And yes it is. Sometimes I just want to do it all myself and be completely independent.

Lesson learned yesterday: Quit trying to figure out everything by yourself. Stop thinking you are so independent. Ask for help when needed. People cannot read your mind so give them a little help. Be thankful for what you can do yourself and be thankful for the many who are more than willing to help if you only ask.

Day 43 - June 9, 2014. To our six children and our fifteen grandchildren we have a message. We know that God lives and that He loves us so much that He sent His Son to die for us so that when we die, we will live again. We are a forever family and will be together again.

When we make mistakes, we can be forgiven. When we hurt, He hurts. When we, your parents, are no longer with you here on earth, we will still live beyond the grave. We will be with our Father in Heaven and we will be together again someday. Death is not the end, but the beginning. Always know how much you are loved and how blessed we are to be family. So while we are all together, hug a little deeper, say I love you a little more often and smile a lot.

Day 44 - June 10, 2014. Yesterday was just one of those days that the stomach and back pain was with Rod most of the day and into the night. My heart hurts for him as he tries so hard to not complain.

Sitting on the deck and feeling the sun helps some. It fills his body with light and warmth. He mentioned how reading the scriptures and praying gives him the same feeling. It fills his soul and body with warmth and light. He said at times he can almost feel God embrace him with love and warmth when he turns his pains over to Him.

A few years ago when Rod had back surgery and the pain was intense, He learned that if he got up and read his scriptures that it almost gave him as much release from pain as it did to take the pain meds. So he started calling his scriptures his pain medication.

Lessons Learned: When all else fails turn your pain and problems over to God. He is the Light that will warm us and will remove the darkness from our life or at least give us enough light that we can see in the darkness of the night.

Day 45 - June 11, 2014. Yesterday was a pretty good day where we had more calm than pain and that made it a great day.

Most of the family from out of town has now returned home and life will return to being a little more quiet and able to get a little more rest when needed, but family will certainly be missed.

Are you comfortable with quiet? I have learned that I was not. There needed to be some noise, even if it was the television, or I needed to be busy doing something all the time. To just sit in silence was just something that made me nervous. It made me think I was being lazy.

I am learning that when someone is in pain, quiet is calming, quiet is healing, quiet is a way to hear the Lord's message He is trying to send to us. I cannot help but wonder why I thought quiet was not okay. I have had some wonderful moments in the quietness of the day and night over the last forty-five days. I have been taught some wonderful lessons in the quiet moments of my life that I hope I never forget.

Lessons Learned: I am learning how to listen to the messages my husband sends without words but in tender looks and smiles. I no longer have to have words to tell me how he feels. I am learning a new language. It is called the language of the unspoken word. It is the language of true love.

Day 46 - June 12, 2014. Yesterday we went to see a pain specialist and she filled us with hope about being able to manage the great pain Rod has been having. So we have high hopes as she changed things around a little and will be ordering a nerve block in his back to help with the pain as well. So we continue to count blessing after blessing and know there are more to come each and every day.

The secret to finding the blessings is to have eyes that are not only looking for them but also expecting to see them. We came home and found a bag of fresh peaches at our door. Thank you, whoever brought it.

Friends brought over a hundred tiny pancakes tonight. On her daughter's social media page, she showed a picture of a tiny pancake her mom had made her after she said she wanted a small one. Her mom has a great sense of humor and gave her what she asked for. I commented on her post that I would like a hundred of them. So she brought them to me tonight. Our family had a lot of fun with those little pancakes and we still have more for tomorrow. Carol I think you could start a side business serving bite size pancakes.

Some of The lessons I have learned over the years about blessings: they don't always look as cute as the hundred little pancakes did. They are often wrapped in packages that have really crummy looking paper and ugly ribbons on them. We sometimes find ourselves saying, *no thank you. I don't really want that blessing. I want one that looks good.*

My Breast cancer in 2003 was wrapped in a really ugly package, but it turned out to be one of my greatest blessings. It taught me more about living and love and laughter than I could have learned any other way.

I could name a few other blessings that were wrapped in really ugly packages also that turned out to be some of my favorite blessings.

May you have a day filled with seeing blessings in your life and if by some chance you don't get one today. Be sure to give one to someone.

Day 47 - June 13, 2014. Another sleepless night for Rod; the night time seems to be the hardest. The pain is less if he sits up and so he tries to sleep sitting up. Not in a chair but on the side of the bed.

An old friend dropped by for a short visit with Rod. What would we do without friends who care? Family helps in many ways including bringing ginger snap cookies. Rod also got a package from a New Jersey friend. It was a homemade sign that simply says what we all feel **WE LOVE RODNEY** with a wonderful note from their family sharing their love for him. It brought tears to his eyes and love into his heart. Being the humble man that he is, he often has a hard time understanding all the love and blessings that keep flowing into our life. To each of you on our journey, we just want you to know how awesome we think you are for taking the time to pray for us and to share your heart with us in so many different ways.

Lessons we are Learning: Love is great. Showing love is greater. The world would be a more wonderful place to live if we made it a daily practice to look around and replace the sadness we see with acts of kindness. There are so many that need it. They may live next door or across the country. Just a note of kindness can change someone's world or even just a smile.

Day 48 - June 14, 2014. I love this quote, "*Don't start your day with broken pieces of yesterday*". It reminds me of my daughter Traci's preschool teacher many years ago. It did not matter what the child did the day before. She always started each kid with a brand new day, with yesterday's behavior in the past.

It also reminds me of my husband and how he is handling his cancer journey. Yesterday may have been a day filled with pain, but each morning when he gets up, it is with a smile and a determined mind that it is a brand new day filled with hope and he moves forward –never backwards.

Day 49 - June 15, 2014. One thing we know for sure; we cannot lean on our own understanding because, if we do, we will certainly see the struggles more than we would like to. But, we can see the bumps as a way to grow and to trust in the Lord.

So for the Dailey's we have chosen to take this journey with the Lord and trust in Him completely. It does not mean we are pain free. It does not mean tears do not escape from our eyes when our thoughts entertain what used to be. It does mean that what the Lord is giving us in this journey is complete trust and faith and that He will embrace us with love and carry us when we are too weak to walk alone.

Yesterday was filled with togetherness, doing things together, being thankful for a wonderful grandson who took care of our lawn, having a great lunch with a son, having a granddaughter come with her parents to give us donuts that she had won for making good grades in school, for watching my husband taking a nap on the deck in a hammock, for watching a movie together at home.

Then as bedtime approached I watched the pain that comes with night time return to my husband and feeling like the war that is raging within his body is like watching a video game going on inside his body as the cancer is at war within his body and is reminding us life is fragile. It is hard to fight a battle when it is all happening in an invisible realm beneath the surface of our reality.

That is when we have to turn it over to God and trust not in our own understanding. Each day brings us greater love for our

Father in Heaven who loves each of us so much that as he helps us over the bumps of life. He shows us beauty that we could never have seen in our busy life that did not allow us to slow down long enough to really see the world as it was meant to be seen.

Day 50 - June 16, 2014. Just a quick one today to let you know Rod did pretty good yesterday. We celebrated Father's Day the week before while all of our kids were in town, but we still had some of our in-town kids over to grill dinner and visit. So thankful for all we have.

May we be blessed to have a spiritual umbrella to carry around when the rain of troubles falls around us to keep us safe and strong.

Day 51 - June 17, 2014. Last night provided a pretty good night's sleep, which is something that we do not see often. Today we visit a pain clinic to set up an appointment for a nerve block which we are hopeful will bring more nights of sleep and rest.

Thank you all for helping us cross a most difficult bridge in our life and being angels to us in so many ways. By the way in case you do not know, we love you; each and every one of you. Be sure and thank the angels in your life today and let them know you love them.

Day 52 - June 18, 2014. Yesterday we went to the Omega Interventional Pain clinic. We were very impressed and felt very hopeful. Yet with anything they do there, there are always risks. We go back this morning and they will do a celiac plexus block, that for most people work to help block pain.

It is a nerve block that blocks the pain signals that would travel up the spine causing the patient to perceive pain. Then he will also start massage therapy next week that not only helps the patient relax but also loosens muscles and relieve muscle spasms. They also sent us home with information concerning an intrathecal pump surgically inserted near the base of the spine to deliver meds and help to decrease potential drug related side effects as the cancer progresses.

Lessons Learned throughout this journey that even though we may not have a cure for his cancer, we may not have to endure so much pain through this journey and for that we are so thankful.

The other lesson I am learning through this is: life in general can be very painful when we suffer in silence trying to solve our own problems our own way. When in reality, we can seek help through the Lord our God and from our friends and family. Our burdens can be so much lighter and so much easier to carry.

When it comes to medical care, there is nothing quick and easy. They did a temporary nerve block on Rod to make sure it works, but it will only last hours to a few days. He has another appointment next Wednesday morning and another appointment to do the three-month block.

I feel like pulling my hair out as I am looking at more bills. All I really want is quick, easy and simple. Is that really asking too much? To be honest, I will settle for all the wonderful prayers you all have been giving for Rod. So thank you for letting me vent and for your many prayers. I feel much better now.

Day 53 - June 19, 2014. I am done pulling my hair out and having a mini breakdown and back to being very thankful for life and all that it offers.

Yesterday was not what I thought it should be, but it served its purpose and we think the block will work and will be waiting patiently to get the real thing instead of the try it version. Rod came home yesterday afternoon and laid down for a nap –four hours. I have not seen him sleep so well in a mighty long time and he slept pretty well last night.

Today is chemo day again. It seems to come so quickly. We are learning to enjoy the people we meet while we are there and to enjoy the day in general. Last week while there we learned about this wonderful handout they had in the front office.

Sometimes great perks come with cancer. So I called the number and learned that because Rod was going through chemo, we can get free house cleaning for ten weeks, two hours each time. They use professionals, and they do all sorts of cleaning. So I called last week and registered and had not heard back from them until yesterday. It will start next week. I also registered for the lawn care. It is every other week until the season ends. We have not heard back from them yet.

Lessons Learned: There are blessings all around us, but many we will never see because we are not looking for them. One of Rodney's favorite verses is "This is the day the Lord made. Let us rejoice and be glad in it.

Day 54 - June 20, 2014. Is life just crazy when you live with cancer? Or is life just crazy when you live?

I think the craziness is just always there when you live a normal life, a sad life, a happy life, a healthy life or a sick life. So we can't think *poor me, if we didn't have this going on in our life everything would be wonderful.*

I am learning to love getting older, because the more I live life, I learn that life is going to be hard, crazy, and wonderful in spite of what is going on.

Yesterday was chemo number five for Rod, and it is amazing when you can actually look forward to going to see a doctor and enter a chemo room with a smile on your face. That is what Rod does.

To be able to laugh and to cry with your doctor is a wonderful feeling; to know that he is not just your doctor but has actually become a friend who really cares about you and how you feel physically and emotionally. We are so blessed to have that in our life.

After Chemo we went to physical therapy to set up appointments for the coming weeks for massage therapy that may help with the back pain. Rod went to these people a few years ago for physical therapy after having had back surgery. They were thrilled to see him after a few years and truly sad when they found out what was going on in his life. This is what happiness is all about; having people in your life who really care about you as a person.

Day 55 - June 21, 2014. We made it through another night of less sleep than we would have liked to have had. Rod fought off a small fever and swollen feet, but the morning has come and a new hope.

Yesterday was a blessed day in many ways. I took Rod to the Temple for a few hours and he loved being there. We have a good friend who does house cleaning part time and she had wanted to give us a gift of service of doing some cleaning for us. Ana, thank you so much for shining clean bathrooms and bedrooms. Your gift was so wonderful.

Lessons Learned in life: You always get more than you give when you give service. It is like paying and tithing to the Lord. You can never out give the Lord. When we give of our time we are always blessed; sometimes right away and sometimes later when you need it most. I am thankful to have been raised by parents who taught by example *Service with love and a smile.*

Day 56 - June 22, 2014. Today is Sunday, my favorite day of the week. When I feel my well is running dry, I can have it refilled each Sunday as I go and have my spirit lifted by those who teach and share their testimony with all that are there.

Sundays are almost like Christmas. There are always spiritual gifts just waiting to be opened, but it is up to us to decide to open them or leave them there. We get to decide how many spiritual gifts we want today. I find that there are as many as I am looking for. What is sad is when I come home with none. It is not because there were not any; it is just that I was not looking. I have also found it to be like a gift exchange. The more I give the more I get back!

Our sons, Terry and Gabe had spent the morning with Rod helping go through things in the garage, tools and things like that for a yard sale next Saturday. They did get a lot done and Rod said he enjoyed having them here. He was in much pain most of the day yesterday and last night. So it was one of those bittersweet days and nights. Too much pain, too little sleep, but we did enjoy sweet talks and feelings of love in our home.

Lessons Learned yesterday: The stuff we thought was so important in life is really just stuff. Little acts of kindness, small moments of peace, wonderful neighbors, long distant friends and family, and faith in our Lord Jesus Christ are the big things. This is what is really important. We are excited to open our spiritual gifts today and hope to be able to give some out also.

Day 57 - June 23, 2014. Yesterday was filled with great lessons learned at church followed by a great visit from Rod's best childhood friend and cousin from Idaho.

The night was our new normal night; pain and more pain, and we are learning to sleep in short naps and to be thankful for what sleep we get, and always look forward to the morning. Rod reminded me this morning as I was starting to work on the update of life at the Dayley's, that he loves and believes in gardens and so did my sister Mary Ann. Some of the happiest hours they spent in life were in a garden. It brings them closer to the Savior as they plant and grow food and flowers.

Lessons I have learned from Rod's garden: He believes in tomorrow, he expects to see the beauty of his garden and he has faith that the seeds he plants will come up and become what they were meant to be.

Rod has a green thumb and helps things to live in his garden. The Savior plants seeds within each of us and then cares for us and delights as he watches us grow into what we were meant to be.

So when we have rainy days in our lives, we must always remember that a garden must have rain and sunshine to grow the seeds that have been planted. I am so thankful for yesterday and for today and for the hope of tomorrows. It takes all three days to help us to grow and become what we are supposed to be.

Day 58 - June 24, 2014. Yesterday was a day filled with kindness, love and beauty. I needed to take Rod in to work for a few hours to his old job at Mercedes so he could do a little training with the guy who is taking over his job. So I thought I would take a good book to read and could not decide which book.

So I took a couple of my old journals. One of them was 1984. How wonderful to read of life's events in 1984. That is the year my life changed for the better for the rest of my life and for all eternity. It was filled with my starting to date Rod Dayley and becoming engaged and married and becoming Mrs. Rodney Dayley.

Last night I was sharing a few pages out of the journal with a very tired husband who was experiencing his nightly pain and as I stopped, he said keep reading, it is such a wonderful story. How thankful I am to have recorded my feelings and my thoughts on how scary it was to let go of your heart and trust in the Lord enough to guide you to true love. If you do not keep a journal, please start today. If you are concerned about what you would say, or think you are not a writer, you will find if you begin, the words will come from your heart and you will fill the pages with things you will forget over the years but as you reread what you have written joy will come into your heart to have recorded your feelings. I now have a record of the beginning of true love to share with my children and grandchildren. What a great gift to leave them.

It is really hard to be sad when our heart is filled everyday with kindness and warmth. We are so very thankful for each of you for taking this journey with us and only pray that your cup of life is filled each day with peace and joy also as we learn what things in life matter most.

Lessons Learned: Record your life's lessons because then you can learn again and again as you reread them. Slow down and enjoy a good book, your book and you will be forever thankful.

Day 59 - June 25, 2014. Yesterday was a day filled with pain but also much needed sleep for Rod most of the day. It is so hard to watch his pain and not be able to fix it. But so thankful that we know prayer changes things.

Lesson learned is: Prayer does not always fix things, but it does change things. For me, it helps me to see more clearly to know that not everything in life has to be fixed right now and sometimes not at all. Sometimes we just need to get out of God's way and let him work His miracles.

Prayer changes the way I feel and the way I act. I am so thankful for prayers, because even though Rod has cancer and still has chemo and pain, he has amazing faith in our Father in Heaven. He still loves his family and friends, he is still thankful each and every day and that, my dear friends is what prayer is all about it.

So here we are on day 59 and we are still happy, we are still finding things to laugh about and cry about and both of us are okay. We have seen so many miracles in the last few months that have nothing to do with cancer, but they have everything to do with people that we care about doing amazing things for others and for themselves.

Day 60 - June 26, 2014. Yesterday was a sunny side up day and I am looking for another one. I worked for about five hours and saw a lot of wonderful friends that stopped by to say hello. And I met a lot of new friends. My day felt a little normal which felt good.

My daughter-in-law, Karen took Rod for his follow up at the nerve clinic and he has an appointment July 9th for the Nerve block that is supposed to last about three months; so we are hopeful. Then my daughter Traci took Rod to his appointment for the deep massage therapy for his back. I am so thankful for so many wonderful kids. Last night we had a huge miracle.

We went to bed at ten and were up at six o'clock this morning with getting up only once for pain meds. In this house that is a really big deal. I have work again today and tomorrow and Rod has chemo at nine thirty and eye doctor appointment this afternoon. Thanks to our son Terry for taking him to those appointments.

Lessons Learned: How good it feels to enjoy a little work and a lot of interaction with old and new friends and accepting help from friends and family is not only okay but needed at times like this. I am learning that I will do all I can do to help myself but It really is not only okay to accept help but also necessary to allow help when it is needed. We wish you all a sunny side up day.

Day 61 - June 27, 2014. This morning Rodney told me that yesterday was filled with tender mercies all day. This was the day he had chemo and an appointment with an eye doctor and his son Terry being his taxi driver. They even came out to my booth at Lehi Days in between appointments and then last night to our grandson, Braden's Arrow of Light in the scouting program. He said everywhere he looked he knew it was a day to rejoice and be glad in it because of seeing all the mercy of the Lord.

Lessons Learned this morning: What I will see today will depend upon the direction I am looking. If I don't like what I am seeing, I can look another way. I have eyes to see mercy and goodness and kindness. However I also need to know the more I give of each of those, the more I will get in return. So what day is it? It is my most favorite day of the week. It is today and it will be the best day ever.

Day 62 - June 28, 2014. Things are just never enough and not what they seemed to be when we first got them. But hidden deep within, we find the greatest joy when we follow our dreams and live the Gospel. Living and being married to a man like Rodney has taught me so much about inner peace and becoming who we should become. I have such inner peace because of lessons I have been taught in life. As we go through this journey, I am still amazed as I see how many lives my husband has touched for good, as more people share their deep love with him for kindness he has done for them, just because he cared.

Lesson Learned: When we let go of our things. We then have room for the really important things in life.

Day 63 - June 29, 2014. Today I look back over the week and look at the time our children invested in their parents. I am amazed at how they pulled this past very busy week together as they made sure we had everything we needed. We ended the week with the yard sale which can drain a healthy person from the energy they need.

Last night Rod and I were tired beyond tired and had nothing left in us. It was almost funny as we struggled to help each other to do things. The yard sale was amazing in sales but also in visiting with friends and newly made friends and we even had a dear friend, Marty that came down from Idaho and stopped and visited. We were so happy to see you, Marty.

Rod will go on Thursday to have the scan done to see if the chemo has done any good on the cancer. It is our hope and prayers that it has slowed it down. We know there is no cure, but our prayers are for a slower moving cancer and making life more comfortable for his very tired body. The following week July 9th will be the nerve block to help with the intense pain also, so we continue to live fully one day at a time and to live with hope of any and all miracles.

Lessons Learned: Remember as a young parent, all those many hours you spent in the car? My daughter even gave me a kitchen magnet many years ago that said Mom's taxi. We took the kids to their activities, and we ran them from one place to another and wondered if we were anything to our kids except transportation.

Now that we are older and in need of help, the role has been reversed. They have become the taxi and the caregivers of not just their kids but also now their parents.

The lesson: Children learn what they are taught and continue to practice what they learned as they become older. What a blessing this has been in our life. Thank You God, for such blessings.

Day 64 - June 30, 2014. Yesterday was a catch up day for much needed rest and also a great church service with two of our youth giving their farewell talks before leaving to be missionaries.

They were both excited to be going and serving the Lord for a couple of years. That was inspiring to hear them share their testimony of serving the Savior. And then it was over to meet with family members for dinner and monthly birthday party! I love being close to our kids and grandkids.

As Rod and I discuss the many different feelings of life in general and also the cancer and what it is doing to his body, we often discuss the past and see it differently now. We see many of our mistakes in the growing up years as mistakes but not something to hold us back but to move us onward and forward as we move closer to the Lord.

It really is true that the pages of yesterday cannot be revised but it is so exciting to know that because of the atonement of Jesus, the pages of today and tomorrow can tell of the many lessons we have learned from our past and we can turn our down days into up days and make our story of life and how we lived one of the most exciting books ever written.

We can take our cancer journey and become as miserable as the pain, or we can take it and be happy in spite of the pain. So we continue every day to look for the blessings, we continue to know there is more good than bad in our lives just as there is in everyone's life.

Lessons Learned: We really can have the life we always dreamed of if we are willing to turn our stumbling blocks into stepping stones that bring us closer to that life. A journal is a great place to put our lessons learned, and years later, as we re-read them, we learn all over again.

Day 65 - July 1, 2014. Yesterday was an early start day, taking Rod to therapy at 8:00 a.m. which was hard for him, since he was awake most of the night trying to sleep sitting up.

But the therapy went well, and when we came home he decided to nap in bed as I ran errands and would periodically come home to check on him.

I was thrilled each time to find him sleeping peacefully without pain and only waking up a few times to eat a little and then fall back asleep. I think his body was in great need of that sleep. Each time I checked on him I had the feeling of peace come over me as well as a deep feeling of love for this wonderful man.

Happiness can be found even in the darkest of times if one only remembers to turn on the light. So as we stumble in the dark we always need to remember the Lord is our light and all we have to do is ask and we can see His brilliance and find great joy in our lives even during a storm or in the darkness of struggles.

For me, each time I checked on Rod and saw him sleeping peacefully, it was if a light was turned on in my soul. A light of hope and faith that God is in charge and will give us the light we need when we need it.

Lesson learned: You can buy lights to plug in so that when your power goes out the lights come on automatically and you are not left in the dark.

We can have lights like that also through our faith in God, so that our love and faith are so strong, that when the darkness comes, our faith shines brightly even in the darkness so we do not have to live in the dark.

Day 66 - July 2, 2014. How many times have we said "someday I will;" Only to learn that sometimes our somedays will be gone or we will not have the health to do what we so passionately wanted to do.

Yesterday was a pretty good day for Rod, but the night was the same; pain and little sleep. The pain was managed most of the day. We spent some time with our grandson, Jared when he showed up to do the yard-work, and also time spent with his mom. It was a quiet day filled with love and time well spent with people we love. The day included a nap for Rod and me; a much needed nap.

There never seems to be enough time for all that should be done, as long as we have time to spend with friends and family and take the time to pray, we always have enough time.

My sister, Mary Ann was always busy, living life to the fullest. She always made time for what was really important including laughter, gardening, taking pictures, traveling and making people feel they were really important. We just knew she would live to be a hundred. Cancer took her from us at age seventy-four while she was still very busy living.

Lessons Learned: It doesn't matter how many clocks you have, and I do have a lot of clocks. It does not mean we have a lot of time. No matter how rich or poor we are, how young or old, we never know how much time we have been given so it is so important to use our time with love and service.

Time is a gift we have all been given. How we spend it is up to us. When we first met with the cancer doctor, he said Rod's cancer was stage-four.

Do you have a bucket list? Start doing the things you always wanted to do but never had time to do, and when you have done those things, do the next things on your list. We both agreed that we have pretty much done the things on our bucket list.

I think this is the advice we should be given when we are born. When you have a burning desire to do something, don't wait until you have stage-four cancer to do it.

What are the things you secretly say to yourself? *Someday I will,* whatever it is, begin now. Now is the time.

Day 67 - July 3, 2014. Yesterday started out hard with a trip to the doctor and then to the hospital for blood work. Rod had a really rough night and his feet and legs are badly swollen. Many years ago he had a foot injury and today water was actually coming out of the twenty year-old stitches of his injury. That was a little freaky.

After close to an hour at the doctor's and having some blood work done, I then took him to his deep massage therapy for his back. He began feeling better and the day improved. And so we continue to tell ourselves good things each day and most of the time we even believe it ourselves.

Today is going to be a great day. Rod has a scan today to determine if the chemo is doing any good at fighting the cancer. If it is, the chemo will continue, if it is not the chemo will stop. Not sure when we will get the results, but I am sure we will get them in the Lord's time.

Lessons I have learned and keep learning: Self-talk is very important. Treat yourself as if you are your very best friend tell yourself good news. I was once asked to teach a class on self-esteem, and I went around the class of thirty-plus women and asked them to tell me just one thing they really liked about themselves. Only about three could comfortably do that. Why can we see so much good about others and not about ourselves?

I encouraged those ladies to look in the mirror each day and tell the person they were looking at how wonderful they are. So if we are going through hard times or good times we really must talk to ourselves in a way that lifts us up because the world is always out there telling us we are not important.

Do not listen to the world, listen to God. He is our Father in Heaven and loves us more than we can even imagine. He wants us to be as kind to ourselves as we are to others. He says in Mark 12:31 "*Love your neighbors as yourself*". Rod and I are not sure what today will bring, but we do know that the Lord will bring us through it.

Day 68 - July 4, 2014. Yesterday morning, Rod had a scan to see if the chemo was working. Yesterday afternoon was his doctor's appointment to get the results.

We are sad to report that the cancer has spread in spite of the chemo, and it has grown in the liver and is now starting to spread to the lungs.

Our doctor felt such sadness as he had to tell us that the chemo was not working and he felt the best care Rod could now have would be in the hands of Hospice.

He suggested the nerve block that was planned for next week was still a good plan to help with relief of the pain of cancer. We will move forward with that and I am sure we will be meeting with Hospice in the coming week and continue our journey but in a different direction.

After we left the doctor's we just drove around and talked and shared our feelings, thoughts and memories. Many of our blessed memories did sneak out of our eyes in the form of tears and sadness. We had many memories that were of laughter, joy and much happiness with which our lives have been filled.

On this wonderful day, as we celebrate the Fourth of July and the freedoms with which we have been blessed to have, we are so thankful that we still live in the land of the free and that we have so many that fight for that freedom still.

Lessons Learned: We still live with cancer, but we also still live with choices of how we will handle the cancer. I love the old saying; *Just when the caterpillar thought the world was over, it became a butterfly.*

We never have to give up hope in miracles, and we will never have to give up looking for and finding blessings in each new day. We will continue the journey and counting each day we are given as a blessing and we will be thankful for an organization such as Hospice whose caring professionals know how to make the journey less painful. We will also be forever thankful for the testimony we carry of knowing that God lives, and He loves us, and His hands are outstretched to bring us back home to Him with much love.

We thank you all each and every day for taking this journey with us, and for giving us your prayers and your encouragement. You have sprinkled our journey with light, hope and joy. Thank you.

Day 69 - July 5, 2014. Last night was normal. The sun goes down and the pain level comes up. The dark comes and the sleep leaves. This morning, sleep and calm find its way into our home once again. So as Rod rests, I share our continued journey with you and pray for a peaceful calm day and night.

As hard as the storms are, it always amazes me how much beauty is in the storm and how much peace we can feel when we know that Heavenly Father is in control.

Our neighbors and doctor came to visit yesterday. It is encouraging when we are blessed with a fine doctor and a good friend and have them be the same person.

We also went to our daughter's and her family for the Fourth of July Dinner. It was such a bitter-sweet time, because yesterday morning their dog of almost thirteen years died and they were sad and we were sad with them. A pet becomes a family member, and it is hard to lose them.

Today we get to go and see our grandson, Jared working on his Eagle Scout project. What a fine young man he is, and we feel honored to have so many great young men and young women that we get to be grandparents to. We continue to count our blessings and we know that today will be filled with them as each day keeps bringing them into our life.

Lessons Learned about my husband: He really is the kind and gentle man that we always thought he was, and he is so filled with kindness and love for his fellowman. As I read the public and private posts to him from yesterday, he was indeed humbled by the outpouring of love from so many of you. Love is a huge dose of medicine for pain relief. So thank you again for being on this journey with us.

Day 70 - July 6, 2014. Saturday was a wonderful day in so many ways. Rod caught up on sleep missed by taking a few naps and we watched a movie at home –such simple, wonderful things.

Of course you probably know today, Sunday, is the best day of the week. It is a day of rest and worship and filling up my heart and spirit to start a new week. For that we are so thankful.

Lessons Learned in inviting others on our journey: We have heard the many private and public messages that you have shared with your heart and your love. We know that love really does grow daily by giving it away to others.

You make it so hard to be depressed or sad because when we count our blessings each day, they always outnumber the sadness. Our hearts are full because of the love of our Savior, our family and our friends. Thank you for expanding the love in our hearts through your caring.

Day 71 - July 7, 2014 Yesterday was such a refreshing day. It had a great balance of rest, worship, family, friends, and feeling gratitude for all my Heavenly Father has done for me and my family.

Rod had his moments of pain, but he also had his moments of joy and happiness. If we could only get the nighttime hours to be good, that would be wonderful.

I am so glad we get to choose how we want to live and how we get to spend the rest of our life. We of course do not always have power over what detours come into our life or what speed bumps we have to cross, but we can choose to see the beauty while on the detour, and we can learn how to avoid as many speed bumps as we can.

I think I need to get a necklace that reminds me that in Heavenly Father's plan there are no true endings; only everlasting beginnings. That is not just a nice thought, it is truth. But in our mind we think of earthly things most of the time. We kind of forget that and think *oh poor me, life is so unfair*.

Last evening our son, Gabe and his family came over to visit. It was such a nice warm feeling, and we were thankful for his wonderful family. Then came another knock on the door, and it was our really sweet neighbor, Stacy carrying fresh baked blueberry-strawberry cobbler, warm and straight from the oven. It was so yummy. Once again, any thought of feeling down just left because you just cannot live with so much kindness and be depressed.

Lessons Learned today: You do not always have to be the receiver of great and thoughtful gifts. You can also be the giver, and then you are blessed even more. So our mission is to discover how to be better givers so we also can bring joy into someone's life. Our hearts have really been overflowing lately with so much gratitude and so very thankful for every one of you on our journey. So we are wishing you a day filled with sunshine and uplifting thoughts. Hugs go out to all of you from the Dayley's.

Day 72 - July 8, 2014. Yesterday was one of our most blessed days. Rod started out with much pain, but it improved quickly and he went for his deep massage therapy for his back which helped so much.

He wanted to go by work at Mercedes for a while and do a little more training with the guy who his taking his place. Then we went out for lunch and ended the day at our son, Terry's home for dinner and a family reunion with Lorie Jo's family. It was so wonderful to visit with her family and know that they have truly become our family as well.

We came home tired but feeling very blessed to have been given such a wonderful day. It ended with Rod being able to sleep in bed instead of sitting up until almost three-thirty this morning. I cannot begin to tell you how wonderful that blessing was for both of us.

We had a few other blessings throughout the day as well. It never ceases to amaze me how we don't always get the blessings we are praying for, but we still get blessings that are just what we need at the moment.

Lessons Learned and relearned: There are some really wonderful people in this world, and when times are a little hard they are more than willing to help make life much easier. I believe this is where sharing our struggles comes into play. When we share what we are going through, it allows people to be creative and come up with ways they can help.

Most of us are not mind readers, and if we do not know what is going on, we assume everything is just fine. Sharing Rod's cancer journey was one of the greatest therapies for the two of us and many of you have shared how it has helped you also. For that we are so thankful because we are each on a journey in this life that is not easy, but that is hopefully made lighter as we share with others.

I have often thought that life is a school where many tests are given, and when we pass enough tests we get to graduate and return back home to Heavenly Father where we hope to hear Him say, "Well done my son or daughter, welcome home." So I think we are eternal students, continuing to live and learn all that we were sent here to learn.

Some of the major subjects we were to learn were love for our fellow man, service to those around us, and learning to turn our problems over to the Lord and trusting Him with our heart, soul and body.

Day 73 - July 9, 2014. What a learning journey this has been. We often feel like a child taking this trip in the body of a grown up. So we therefore know that faith is taking the first step even when we don't see the whole staircase.

I often think of the song I am a Child of God, and we all are at any age. Yesterday morning was filled with great pain for Rod. It is unbelievable what cancer can do to the inside of a body. Even though it has the power to take a body, we still fight to keep it from taking our spirit and our love of life and living.

Today was the day Rod was supposed to have the nerve bock to help manage the pain, and we have been looking forward to it.

Yesterday they asked if he was on antibiotics and we said *yes* (he has an infection in his stomach,) so he has another six days on them. We learned that he has to be off of them for ten days before they could do the block.

We were not really happy about that, and the child comes out in you when you are not really happy about something, so we pouted for a few minutes, and then realized that does not do us any good. So we will turn it over to the Lord and continue down the learning journey.

Lesson learned: Read every detail on those papers the doctor gives you; it was all there in black and white, and if you can't change something don't let it change who you are. Just accept it and keep on moving.

So today will still be a good day. We still meet with the doctor and that will help us with Hospice and we will find many more blessings today on this learning journey.

I am including the words to I am a Child of God in case some of you do not know the song.

I am a child of God, and he has sent me here,
Has given me an earthly home, with parents kind and dear.
Lead me, guide me, walk beside me, help me find the way.
Teach me all that I must do, to live with him someday
I am a child of God, and so my needs are great;
Help me to understand his words, before it grows too late.
I am a child of God. Rich blessings are in store;
If I but learn to do his will, I'll live with him once more.

Day 74 - July 10, 2014. If the plan is not working, who would have thought you could just change it?

Yesterday we were so disappointed about not being able to get the nerve block. Little did we know that there was a bigger plan. We went to talk to the palliative doctor (one who knows everything about managing pain.) We thought we would be talking about Hospice, but there was a bigger plan that we knew nothing about.

My husband was there with the same doctor a month ago and his weight then was 148 pounds. Yesterday it was 172 pounds. Remember the swelling in the legs? It is also in the stomach and it has a name; *ascites.* That is when pancreatic cancer has spread to the tissues in the abdominal lining. It can be treated through a procedure called *paracentesis*, which is scheduled for today. The procedure cannot be done if you are on Hospice.

Our doctor called the other doctor to do the nerve block and it looks like that now may happen much sooner than they had told us. Neither one of these things could be done had we been on Hospice. So Hospice is on hold, but hope is looking brighter for pain relief. Who would have thought we could continue to learn so much on this journey? Yesterday was a wonderful day, and we went to bed at nine-thirty and slept until four-thirty this morning.

If you are wondering if your prayers are working; the answer is a very big *yes*! We continue to see miracles and blessings each and every day. Thank you so much.

Our new palliative doctor also made changes in meds that are sounding promising. So we start this day with much excitement and hope for more relief of pain.

Lessons Learned: Just because we are on a roller coaster of emotional pain does not mean we have to stay there. Sometimes, we can find the help we need to get off the roller coaster. We do not have to assume that if our plan is not working to reach our goals, we have failed.

There just may be other ways to reach our goal that we have not thought of. So we pray more, we continue to search for answers we do not have and trust that the Lord hears our prayers and brings us answers we knew nothing about. God can move mountains, if we believe.

If anyone wants some great information about palliative care in pancreatic cancer go to *www.cancercouncil.com.au/wp-content/uploads/2014/05/UC-Palliative-Care-CAN486.pdf.* Knowledge is power.

Day 75 - July 11, 2014. If I were to create a plaque that summarized my feelings today, it would simply say, **BLESSED BEYOND BELIEF.** Those are the words that are constantly in our hearts on this journey of life.

Before I tell you about yesterday, I must tell you how very grateful Rod and I are for the life we have been given. How very grateful we are for our family and for friends that lift us up and most of all for the love of a Heavenly Father who has carried us over many difficult times in our lives and has given us just what we needed when we needed it the most. We truly are blessed beyond belief and eternally grateful for the life we have been given.

Yesterday we had an appointment at the hospital for them to remove liquid from around Rod's liver which was putting pressure on the lungs and liver, making it difficult to breathe. They let me sit in and watch while they did this.

They removed two liters of liquid. It is amazing what can be done to make life easier. This was a blessing to us. Then while at the hospital we got a call from the doctor's office that will do the nerve block, and they have decided they can do the procedure sooner. Monday afternoon we have an appointment for that blessing.

As you may know, Rod and I always start our day looking for blessings. It's like a treasure hunt for us to see how many blessings we can find. We never end our day without having spotted quite a few.

Lessons Learned: Have you ever done word search puzzles? You are given the words, but then you get to search and find them. For me, it's so hard to find some of those words, but they are always there. All we have to do is locate and circle them. Once they are found, I'm amazed that I didn't see them before.

It's the same when we play the game of searching for blessings. There they are right before our eyes, but sometimes a little difficult to see until we find them, and then we wonder why it took so long to see them. May we all enjoy our blessing search game today. Find them and embrace them in our hearts so others may see them also.

Day 76 - July 12, 2014. Good morning. Most of Rod's day was good yesterday until about four-thirty, and the pain killers could not seem to touch the stomach pain for many hours. Yet he continued to be strong. I am not sure if the pain pills finally kicked in later in the night or if it was just exhaustion, but he was finally able to get some sleep after one o'clock in the morning.

When I met Rod in 1983, I was impressed with how strong he was in the Gospel. His testimony was strong and solid and it has continued to grow. Life has not been perfect, and we have had set-backs with job losses and health problems, etc. But it never shook his testimony. I am so thankful to be married to such a man of great faith.

Lesson learned: Life does not have to be perfect to have a perfect faith in God. Life may be hard but it does not have to make us hard. There is always a rainbow at the end of a storm, and life continues with the help of the Savior if we continue to be strong in the Gospel.

Day 77 - July 13, 2014. Sometimes we just simply need someone to be there to care. Do we not all feel this way?

Yesterday was a wonderful day filled with having breakfast with Rod's baby brother, Stacy, from Idaho and wonderful wife and daughter and then a nice long visit. So the morning was filled with growing up memories between two brothers and lasted until almost noon when the pain decided to visit again.

Rod would get some rest and a good nap. In the afternoon he got to enjoy a visit with our son, Terry and after that just a nice mellow quiet day and evening.

As we share this journey just remember, it is more than enough just to know you are there, to see a comment, or just a *like* by your name helps us to know that we are cared about, and that is more than enough.

As the days are passing, Rod finds it more difficult to do what he once did, but he has said over and over again, "It is completely in the Lord's hands, and it will be alright. I have found that each morning he finds great joy in the writings of this journey, and the wonderful responses. So please know he always smiles as I read them to him.

Lessons Learned: When someone has cancer and you do not know what to say – it's okay. A smile or a hug work really well also. Sometimes just the words *I care* go a long way.

Most of you know that I am a breast cancer survivor of eleven years. I have been with Avon for over twenty years, and often in my work we do a breast cancer awareness table at many events. You would be surprised how many people will go out of their way so as not to pass our table.

Cancer is a scary word. But talking to people about it will not mean you are going to catch it. Then there are others who have been touched by cancer or had family members touched, and they are the first to come up and talk to us and share their story.

People grow so much from bad experiences. Cancer usually does not mean you are going to die. It just means you are going to change the way you live and look at life. When we share our life with someone who is hurting in any way, it can change our own life for the better for the rest of our life. I wish you a wonderful day of worship.

Day 78 - July 14, 2014. Yesterday was a day of rest and pain for Rod most of the day. He had hoped to go to church but just could not get his body to work with him. So he did get a lot of sleep which he has been missing since cancer has been taking over his body.

It was good that he could sleep. Hopefully he has the rest he needs to have the nerve block this afternoon at three o'clock and maybe, just maybe, we will be able to see some good changes in the pain level in his body.

Regardless of what does or does not happen, we have been blessed to have the key to happiness in our life and that key is learning to love the Lord our God, and obey Him, and commit our self firmly to Him. This is the key to life.

I have been reading a book and there was a part that caught my attention about a homeless man and a rich man talking about the keys on the rich man's key ring.

The homeless man said *"I know it ain't none of my business, but does you own somethin that each one of them keys fits?"*

The rich man glanced at the ten keys on his ring, and said "I suppose" The homeless man said "Are you sure you own them, or does they own you?"

This made me think about all the things I own, and have often wondered if I owned them or if they owned me. I am grateful to know that at least one of the keys I own is the key of faith in my Father in Heaven, and that is the key I treasure most.

Lessons Learned today: I can not do anything in life by myself. With the Lord's help, I can do small things, with great love. I get to wrap my husband's legs every morning with ace bandages to help with the swelling, and then each night, I get to un-wrap them.

I told Rod as I was un-wrapping them that it was just like un-wrapping a package every night. He looked at me and said "Do you really feel that way?" And I said "yes, I do. If it was reversed, wouldn't you feel that way?" He admitted he would.

So is that a big thing? No, and it does not have to be a big thing to show love. We can do that by little things. I have another example, Connie, thank you for bringing over the three yummy cookies for us tonight. It was a small thing to her, a huge thing to us.

Day 79 - July 15, 2014. Family time holds so many memories and we are so thankful for every memory we have made over the last thirty years with each other and with our children and grandchildren.

Yesterday was one of our days of hope. Rod had the nerve block done. As of this morning it does not appear to have worked. Last night was filled with much pain once again and little sleep. But we are thankful that he tried the chemo and the nerve block, because we will not have to wonder *"What if it would have worked?"*

We will continue to hope and to pray, but we are at peace in turning our time into God's hands. We are so very thankful for His love and for the wonderful family and friends he has blessed us with on our journey.

We will continue to walk with our hands in His, and He will guide and direct us. We will continue to look for new blessings each and every day and I can almost promise you that they will be there.

Lesson Learned: Family time brings us closer to God when we are together or when we are reliving the moments we spent together. Dear friends have become a huge part of our family and we cherish that time also.

Day 80 - July 16, 2014. What a difference a day brings. I know you keep hearing this from me. Why am I always so forgetful to remember just because yesterday did not bring us the peace we had hoped for does not mean tomorrow will not be just what the doctor ordered.

Yesterday was better than the night before, and we even did a few normal things without pain being at the scale of a seven or eight. Many of you posted yesterday that maybe it needed more time to work, and that brought us hope. Some even said it may take days. So we are looking for that delayed gift.

We also had several visitors; thank you for coming by and that always makes the day wonderful. Not to mention a really sweet neighbor that brought us a treat.

Rod and I are spending more time talking about old memories, old friends, new memories and new friends, and each time it makes us smile and it warms our heart. We take the time to find humor and time to laugh.

I love it when Rodney tells jokes and makes people laugh. Just because today may not be what we wanted does not mean each day will be bad.

It always amazes me how many times some people are angry or mad so often that you would think there was a reward for those feelings. My Mom used to get mad at my dad every now and then, and she would say *sometimes I was mad so long I would forget what I was even mad about.*

They were married sixty-seven years. Good, clean humor to me is like a breath of fresh air. My sisters and I used to laugh so hard we could not even remember why we were laughing. We were so thankful for things that made us laugh.

Lessons Learned: Share laughter, it is great medicine. It makes your heart feel good and lightens your burdens. I love to see smiles on peoples' faces; it means someone fun is at home inside that body. Assignment for today for each of us is to smile at ten or more people. It may be the only smile they see today.

Day 81 - July 17, 2014. As Rodney's body grows weaker, I do believe his spirit grows stronger. I am in awe of how strong he is in his faith and love of our Father in Heaven.

Yesterday, our doctor said it was time to get him onto Hospice because there are great resources there that can help him in so many ways. They will come and meet with us today.

Yesterday we made final plans and payment for the funeral of not only Rod's but mine and Diani's also so that now we do not have to think about that again.

The other day we got the headstone for the three of us designed so they can start working on it. It's a bench, so if you want to come and chat, you will have a place to sit. We already had our plots in the lovely Lehi cemetery which is just a little over a mile from our home.

We even went by our favorite florist and looked at flowers, and then Rod spent time working on the funeral program and who he wants to speak, sing and pray.

I want you to know it was one of our best days yet. It was full of peace, love, laughter and a very strong spirit. It was not a sad day.

I asked him yesterday afternoon after a very full day what his pain level was, and it was only a one or two. Mine was a three or four – just kidding. I think his nerve block is starting to work. I am more in love with this man than I have ever been. I look forward to spending an eternity with him.

Lesson Learned: Never measure a person's strength by what you see. Some of the strongest people I know have a little trouble getting around and may need a little extra help. That only means their body is weak, and we are not our body. We are our spirit, our mind, our heart and our soul, and that can be stronger than anything.

Day 82 - July 18, 2014. What would our life be like if we trusted that we are always being guided? Yesterday was one of those days when you felt like you were watching a movie that was sweet but kinda sad. And then you realize that the stars of this movie are your husband and yourself.

At home and being introduced to Hospice Care that is for someone who has been given less than six months left to live. It all becomes real that your life is really changing and the life you had is not going to be the same.

The sadness is there, but so is the beauty because you are not alone and you have caring people you have just met that entered your life to make your husband and you more comfortable on this journey and you discovered how blessed you are once again.

The Lord has not left us alone because we have God; we have each other and our children and grandchildren. We have all of you who are traveling on this journey with us, and now we have a team of people who are trained to not cure you but care for you and help you make all the changes with knowledge and care and comfort.

Thank you, dear Father in Heaven for another tender mercy. The Hospital bed is small and is harder for Rod to be comfortable in. But at least it is at home and in our bedroom instead of a hospital. He was actually up only twice last night and slept pretty well.

Last night the swelling in his feet and legs was bad, but with his feet elevated through the night, the swelling went away and he had skinny legs again this morning. Now to find the secret to keeping them down; we wrap them first thing in the morning.

Lessons Learned: God really is guiding us along our road of life. He is helping us to make choices that will shape us and help us become who we were sent here to be. Also, because He is constantly guiding us, we have what we think are accidental blessings in our lives, as we see someone we have not seen in years, just because we are at the same place at the same time.

I do not believe they are accidents, but gifts from a loving Heavenly Father who wants to give us an extra gift that day. May we each be blessed today to see and recognize the many gifts He has for us today.

Day 83 - July 19, 2014 Yesterday was another day together so therefore it was a good day. We know that when we get up in the morning there will be some bumps in the road. We know we will hit a few walls and even stumble a few times –so what? We do not let that determine whether or not we will be happy.

We really are able to condition our circumstances instead of being conditioned by them. It is seldom easy, but it is always possible if we practice a lot. We have some very dear friends that took Diani for a fun weekend of camping, hiking, movies, church and dinner, and she has been excited all week. It is so wonderful when she can get a little break from reality. So thank you Katie and Jonica.

There is so much kindness in the world and we have been touched by a lot of it. We will never be able to say thank you to all of you and so many more who are not even on social media for your random acts of kindness and offers and acts of service. We love you and thank you.

Lessons we continue to learn: Life is awesome. Living is a joy. Sharing your journey, what ever it may be always opens the door to allow others to open the door into their life also. When the doors are open, that is when we really get to know one another and learn to care.

Day 84 - July 20, 2014. Last night was a tough one, but filled with love and help from our kids. Rod fell in the bathroom, and I could not help him up, so I called our son, and he and his wife came over after eleven o'clock that night and helped to get him into bed.

Cancer robs the body of strength and the ability to get up sometimes. But the sweetness of our kids and the deep love they have for their dad is such an amazing gift. We are so very thankful to have family that cares about family. So for now we will keep calm and pretend this is part of our earthly lesson.

Lesson learned: Call for help when you need it, and the giver and the receiver will both be blessed. Also remember that all of life is a lesson and sometimes tests follow the lessons, and we will do much better if we can keep a sense of humor, a ton of love in our heart and stay calm.

Day 85 - July 21, 2014. Sunday was not our normal Sunday. We did not go to church, but we watched some great church programs on television and watched the Spoken Word at nine thirty that morning. We have gone several times to see that in person and love it every time. We love listening to the Mormon Tabernacle Choir.

Rod spent most of his day sleeping in his new power-lift recliner chair we got on Saturday, and it gives him a new freedom. He can get out of the chair by himself, and it reclines nicely so he can get a good nap without being in bed.

Diani came home from a wonderful weekend with her friends; it was so wonderful that they made her weekend so wonderful. Rod is growing weaker quicker than I like, but every now and then, we still see a smile and a twinkle in his eye and hear a laugh. That is music to my ears and to our family also.

I wish I understood how a man having a blast at Disney World in February with Diani and me and our Avon friends, and then walking on the beach in Mexico in April and having much more energy than I did, can be told on April twenty-eighth that he has pancreatic cancer stage four.

I really do not understand. But, I really do not have to, because Heavenly Father understands, and I know that I cannot take one day for granted.

We never know when it will be time to prepare for a new journey. The wonderful thing about Rodney is he has lived prepared for years. That makes the journey so much easier. One thing we know for sure. There is always something to be thankful for.

Lessons Learned: Most lessons are learned by living real life. We hurt some of the time and learn that when we survive our hurts we grow stronger each time, and it gives us courage the next time a problem pops up.

I never had to go through any of my major problems alone because God was always right there lifting me when I really just wanted to pull the covers over my head. I would wake up the next morning and hear the birds singing and knew life was going on with or without me and deciding I might as well move forward because there was more for me to do and to learn.

Day 86 - July 22, 2014. My dear husband spent much time sleeping today. Hospice angels came this afternoon; first the social worker and later the nurse.

They were able to get an appointment set up for this morning for a drain to be put in so as his body fills up with fluid around his liver and lungs we can drain it, we are so thankful for how quickly Hospice can get things done.

The Nurse will come back this afternoon to check on him and make sure all is well. I am so hoping that this will make a difference for him to be able to be more comfortable.

He said such a sweet and tender prayer before we retired to bed last night. I am constantly touched and amazed at his love for Our Father in Heaven, his family and his friends.

We both want you all to be aware that we know that we are children of God. When we come to that knowledge, we know that He will guide us and walk beside us through out our life time. He helps us to know we never have to settle for being anything but our best self.

Lesson learned: When God is your Father in Heaven, it makes it much easier to walk tall and to always rise above the ordinary. It certainly does not mean we are better than others.

It does mean we are all pretty special, and we get to be brothers and sisters with everyone we meet; because they too are children of God. Rod and I are so blessed to have so many of our brothers and sisters taking this journey with us and we are forever grateful.

Day 87 - July 23, 2014. Have you ever wondered what angels look like? I just wanted to share word pictures of a few human angels that entered our life yesterday. I wish I had taken more pictures of others and then of course the many angels that we cannot see but feel, seemed to be present yesterday also.

Yesterday was a hard day with much pain, but a doctor and the hospice nurses performed miracles in getting Rod into out-patient for the drain surgery he needed and it went well.

Thanks go out to a great son for driving us and waiting with us, leaving another great son at home to start the construction of a wheel chair ramp needed to be built in the garage to give Rod more freedom.

Some of our sons and grand sons worked hard to perform that miracle, and then the Hospice nurses spent hours at our home helping Rod to manage the pain. They got him a pain pump which is working wonders already.

Earlier in the day we had some good friends bring us ears of corn and followed by three neighborhood angels who visited us once again with goodies and a lovely note.

Just the night before, I called a dear friend to voice my concerns and fears, and I was feeling very helpless on how to best help Rod on this journey. How wonderful to have friends who will help ease your mind when it is running a little crazy.

Lesson learned: *Hebrews 13:2 out of the New Testament: Be not forgetful to entertain strangers: for thereby some have entertained angels unawares.*

My lesson learned was that strangers, friends, family, neighbors, everyone we come in contact just could be and perhaps often are angels in our life who help us believe in miracles all over again.

How important it is that we too wear angel shoes so that we may also help someone believe in miracles again. Who will you be an angel to today?

Day 88 - July 24, 2014. Yesterday began with a visit from Rod's cousin, Rex, from Idaho who was his best friend growing up and his wonderful wife Nancy. What a delightful way to start the day.

Later in the day a visit from one of Rod's good friends, who just stopped to check on him and ending the night with one of the sweet families in our neighborhood just checking on him and bringing sea shells from their vacation.

They brought two of their daughters and one had written her sweet testimony of the Gospel to share with Rod. She left the written copy with him.

Visits, calls and social media messages are things he looks forward to. However, if you visit, just know he may take a little nap while your here. It's the meds and the cancer that wear him out –not you.

The Hospice nurses and helpers continue to assist us through this journey and the Gospel helps us to better understand the process also. As we begin the journey, things seem kind of normal, just a little different, and as time passes, they seem to have one foot here with us and the other foot half way to heaven.

It starts to seem a little lonely even while they are still here because they are no longer here full time. They are preparing for the trip back to Heavenly Father.

I am so thankful to know the trip he is taking and that each of us will take when it is our turn is one that we have been preparing for our whole life.

It is more wonderful to return to live with our Heavenly Father than we can even imagine. But, while we live here on earth with our earthly brain, it is still hard to let go.

The other night I told Rod, he must feel like a wishbone being stretched, because I am on this side pulling to keep him here, and God is on the other side pulling and saying, *it's almost time.* He looked at both arms and said, *No stretch marks yet.* So maybe I get to keep him a little longer.

Lesson learned: We think our thoughts, we feel our thoughts, but, if we do not write them down we seldom remember our thoughts.

Toba Beta said, *Send message to the future by writing it down today.* So to me this says if you want your children and grandchildren to really know who you are and what you believe, better get that pen and paper out and write it. This is how we can live forever in our loved ones' hearts.

Day 89 - July 25, 2014. This morning Rod woke up around four o'clock and was very confused. He has several tubes attached to him and his legs are too weak to walk so that adds to the confusion. He is now, an hour later, resting once again. I'm feeling helpless on the best way to help him. The Hospice nurse will be here this morning. I am so thankful for those who understand this process and help me to better understand.

Yesterday was another day of learning and growing. I am so thankful for Hospice nurses. I think they must be angels with hidden wings. They help the patient and they also care for the family.

Even though it was another day with much confusion, it was also a day of a wonderful visit with dear friends from New Jersey which have now moved to Ohio and it has been too long since we have seen them.

Amy and Neal, thank you both so much for coming to visit while you were in Utah, and also for being checked on by family members with love and concern and cleaning window wells and the garage.

Gabe took his dad out to the garden where some weeding and harvesting took place. As I took their picture, I remembered Gabe's baptism which took place shortly after Rod and I got married in 1984, and I stand amazed at how time has gone so quickly.

I am so happy that our children still ask their dad for advice and counsel. Each of our children really has learned how to plant seeds of kindness and harvest a garden of love where ever they go.

Lesson learned: The greatest gift is love, and the gift of giving yourself to those you love and serve. The easiest gift is money, and things you can wrap in paper. But love is the greatest of all gifts. Real love for friends or family is so hard to describe. But it has a way of bringing inner peace and calm to our soul.

The beauty of the gift of love is we never have to lose it. It goes beyond the grave into eternity.

Day 90 - July 26, 2014. Yesterday was touch and go, but finished with a wheel chair ride around the neighborhood with two of our sons pushing him and stopping to chat with his angel friends the Packer's. Then it was home to crash and fall into bed. Our son Terry spent the night, and I slept downstairs to a full nights sleep. I actually slept in, so my post is a little later than normal.

I have never been on a roller coaster at the fair; number one, because I am chicken and number two, because I am scared of heights. So as a gift Heavenly Father gave me a roller coaster ride in real life many times, and I have learned the through the best of times or the worst of the times, our Father in Heaven is always with us.

Hospice gives you a book letting you know some of the signs that the time is getting close for your loved one to be leaving you, and yesterday was one of those days that many of those signs were present.

So emotionally, it was a very bitter sweet day. Also a big thank you goes to the Larsen family for the yummy lemon cake.

Lesson Learned: The biggest lesson I learned over again was *Let go and let God.* He is in charge, always has been, and always will be. He gave us a wonderful ending to an emotional day.

Also, He will give us such a wonderful ending on earth and a wonderful beginning as we enter Heaven when we have finished our work on earth.

Day 91 - July 27, 2014. Brings a gathering of family to be close by for a little while as things become more difficult, we bond together and help bless Rod by his being surrounded by the love of his family.

Thank you to our children that live here for helping out so much and feeling the thrill of serving a man who has spent his life serving his children and family members. Thank you to McKay for driving out from California and Shelley for driving out from Boise.

All six kids will be together for a short time once again. Shelley, thanks for stopping by Burley and bringing Rod's brother, Kevin. Yesterday was a day of quiet and not so quiet excitement once again. That is our new normal and we are thankful to have it.

Lessons Learned: People come in and go out of our lives throughout our lifetime. Family is always there in good and hard times. So the family really is one of God's masterpieces. I love the way we are all different and yet you put us all together and you have the complete picture of what a happy family looks like.

Day 92 - July 28, 2014. Yesterday morning, my daughter and I had a nice visit with the Hospice nurse after she checked Rod's vitals. She talked to us in another room about what is going on with his body.

He is very close to the final stages of his life here on earth and he is preparing to return home to Heavenly Father. Since we are not in charge but God is, it will all be according to God's time table and not ours.

So we will enjoy serving Rod, and helping him to be as comfortable as possible. It has truly been a joy and delight to be able to serve this extremely wonderful husband and father and friend.

Our family is so thankful for the great love of Our Father in Heaven, and so thankful that Rod Dayley has given us love and patience and kindness throughout the years.

We thank each of you who have traveled this journey with us and have played a very important part in this journey.

We are sad to have Him leave early, but our hearts are full of joy and blessings for everything he has brought into our lives which will stay with us into eternity and we know that he will never be very far away. Our children made it here safe and sound yesterday and for that we are thankful.

Lesson learned: Cancer is a gift; I choke as I write this because it is hard to see it as a gift. When Rod was told he had stage-four cancer and that he would probably live two to six months, he told us that cancer is a gift.

It has given us ninety-two days and counting to grow closer to each other and to see what is really important in life. He was able to plan his own funeral and choose the way he would want things done. He has been able to say *I love you* over and over again and so have we.

So the lesson is when we are given something we really do not see as a gift, look at it more closely, because it just may change our lives and help us to live them even better than before. God's timetable is what it is because He sees the big picture. We only see with our earthly eyes.

Day 93 - July 29, 2014. I have no idea how to describe yesterday, but I will give it a try. Rod is still with us in body, but he spent the day and night quietly talking and it was seldom to us.

I suppose when you are getting ready for such a big trip to Heaven, it requires a lot of energy. There is very little time for things like food and drink; certainly no time for television or small chit chat.

He was focused most of the day seeing things I could not see and discussing things I could not hear. It almost felt like I was on sacred ground and it was a wonderful feeling.

We had decided to have family all together last night and have a special prayer and priesthood blessing said for Rod by our son, Terry, to let him know that when God was ready to call him home that it was okay to go.

It was a prayer given to release him from his earthly duties so that he could return to our Father in Heaven, in peace knowing that he had done all that was required of him here.

When the prayer was finished, Rod who had not really spoken to us all day, quietly said *Thank you,* and then we were each able to quietly tell him how much we loved him and would miss him.

I know this will sound strange to many, but it was filled with tears and sadness and yet with so much love and peace and joy in our hearts. We feel that we and Rod are ready when the time comes and we are in no hurry.

Lesson learned: My son, Gabe shared this thought with me by Dr. Seuss: *So we don't cry because it's over, because we are an eternal family, and it is not over,* (Poor Doctor Seuss must not have understood that) but we do smile because it happened and we will be together again for all time and all eternity.

Always thankful, Joyce Dayley

Day 93 - Continued - July 29, 2014. Rodney McKay Dayley is now at peace, as he walked through the open door to be with Heavenly Father this morning around six forty-five. He is now at rest and has the peace he was hoping for.

I will write again in a few days when I know what the arrangements are. Again we both thank you all for taking this journey with us. It has now been completed. May God bless you with peace and love today.

§

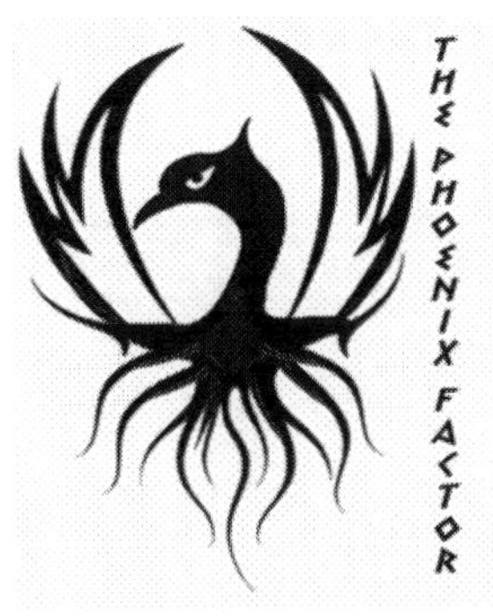

Mike. The end of something very special is always sad, no matter how much joy it includes. This story certainly contains sorrow, pain, grief, and uncertainty, but it also contains hope, trust, and love. In a way, it is the end of one thing and the beginning of another.

I never met Rodney or Joyce Dayley, but I feel like I know them both intimately. I consider them as friends and almost family. You cannot share the depths of your soul with others without forming an eternal bond.

I am confident that Joyce will continue journaling her life and will leave a rich legacy of valuable treasures for those who will read them.

This journal contains a powerful message of a more powerful peace in the lives of an entire family. As Day 93 drew closer with the passing of each preceding day, there was no notable increase in angst, overwhelming sorrow, or debilitating fear of the inevitable.

Of course, Joyce and Rodney's family did not know when the last day would be, and that proved to be a blessing. Rodney lived a full life until the end of his life.

I am sure that when the time came for Rodney to go home, he did so with confidence and a smile of wonderful expectation on his face. I am also sure that as Joyce experienced his departure, the Heavenly Father touched her spirit with the warmth of His love and assurance that all was well.

§§§

Chapter Sixteen

Lady with the Rosary – Patricia (Trish) Gurney

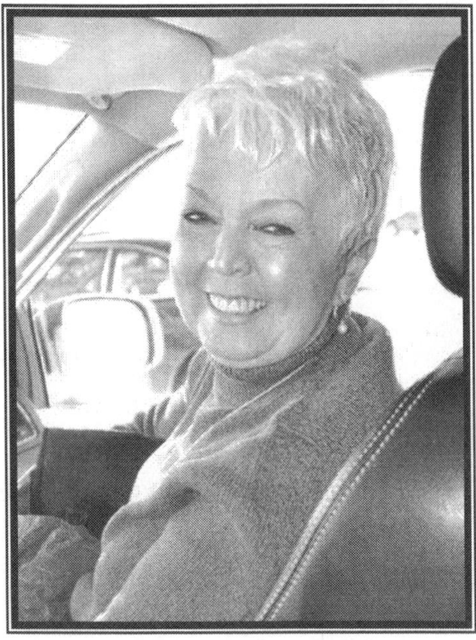

I believe it was during my second round of chemotherapy as I sat in the infusion room just thinking and observing the other patients.

They all appeared to be in different stages of discomfort, weakness, agony, or just being very cold and trying to stay or get warm.

Some patients wore coats, boots, hoodies, and others used blankets. Others seemed un-bothered by what they were going through.

Some folks visited with friends and family, some obviously wanted privacy, some read while others used electronic devices to help them while away the hours spent in treatment.

As a writer myself, I am always interested in the title of the books that cancer patients read. Older folks seem to prefer faith oriented books, romance novels appear to be in vogue with ladies, and the younger ones usually use the electronic readers, so I can't tell what they like. I do know from being a grandfather, that zombies and vampires oftentimes top the charts.

On this particular day, I noticed a mature lady sitting with a nice looking young man and seemed to be chatting about whatever. She was also grasping a Rosary.

Being a former Catholic, I recognize the methods Catholics employ when they pray. The Rosary is a very important and sacred aid to prayer. Devotion to the rosary is one of the most notable features of popular Catholic spirituality.

Pope John Paul II placed the rosary at the very center of Christian spirituality and said that it was *"among the finest and most praiseworthy traditions of Christian contemplation."*

This lady would become my friend as the days passed and we shared infusion times. She was very positive, and manifested a pleasant demeanor that was contagious and certainly brightened my day as I journeyed deeper into the throes of the treatments.

We began our relationship when I introduced myself to her and her son. I explained that if she had not already read Lynn Eib's book, When God & Cancer Meet, I wanted to give her one as a gift, and offered to pray with her.

I detected hesitancy as she mentally and spiritually processed this Protestant man's offer to pray with her. After I further explained that I was a former Catholic; she asked me a couple of theological questions, such as how I felt about Purgatory and such. I guess I passed the test, and we became prayer partners and friends.

I could tell as we sat together that she was under physical stress with the treatments that grew in intensity and were changed periodically to meet the changing challenges of the disease. You would never know it by her attitude. She was happy, outgoing, talkative, and pleasant with a testimony about her Lord that was over the top.

I would discover as our relationship grew, that she prayed for many things including her family and others with cancer and that she had placed all her trust in God regarding her own cancer.

In my personal experience, and those of others that I have researched, people look for and need personal testimonies of victories, fears, failures, and ultimate redemption from the grasp of this fearful thing called cancer. They also need friends and family to accept them as they are, cancer included.

Those of us who have walked the dark vale of cancer and treatments know too well the sadness that wells up inside of us when someone stares at us and walks away or obviously keeps their distance when they observe our presence.

We realize that there are many folks who just cannot deal with cancer or various significant diseases in others. But understanding their hesitation to associate with us doesn't make it any easier to deal with.

Seventy-one year old Patricia (Trish) Gurney drives a car and most of the time when she has the energy, gets around very well. She not only has, but shares a personal testimony with anyone interested in listening. Trish has two sons, forty-four year old

John Charles Gurney, who lives locally, and forty-nine year-old Michael Joseph Gurney, who lives in Virginia.

Hers is a story worth telling; in part because from the beginning, she expected never to be cured of cancer (as we say), but she had hope. I am talking about the kind of hope that can be experienced only by those who sincerely believe that their fate rests in the hands of a loving and powerful God.

She was informed in July that she would be in treatment for the remainder of her life, however long that might be. Two years ago, Trish was diagnosed with colon cancer, stage three and shortly thereafter was diagnosed with colon cancer of the liver. As Trish spoke to me, she did so in a very matter of fact manner.

§

Trish. I remember with each diagnosis that I never cried, nor did I panic. I told God that I loved Him and that I was all right with the cancer I had inside of me. From that time on, I have felt His presence with me in a very special way. This is especially important because my doctors would not give me a prognosis of how much time I had left to live.

§

Mike. I have found that most cancer survivors share a vision of one day being told by their oncologist that they are cancer-free. They endure the treatments in hopes that one day they will be finished with not only the treatments but the disease. So what is the mind-set of one who knows she will never experience that freedom?

Trish says that she lives from scan to scan, one treatment to the next, one day at a time. Her medication changes as the cancer evolves or reacts to her current treatments. Chemotherapy is her constant companion along with the side effects. CAT Scans, PET Scans, tests to make sure that the cancer cells are not gaining strength from her blood, infusions, and blood tests would be a part of her life for the rest of her tenuous life.

Trish has been a medical treatment trooper for many years. When she was thirteen years old she was a patient in a Catholic cardiac hospital where she was bed-ridden for a year with active rheumatic fever. In 1988 she had two separate operations to treat brain aneurysms from which she still carries the scars and soft spots in the sides of her head. Again, she said to me.

§

Trish. I remember seeing my surgeon come into my room wearing a *Jesus First* pin on his lapel. He prayed aloud with me, and I immediately knew I was in God's hands. I said to God, "I love you and it's all right that I have these things in my head."

I accepted what was happening to me. I remember thinking how an aneurysm could burst with the slightest movement of my head. That was when I surrendered everything to Him.

§

Mike. From the time she was a small child for thirty years, Trish could not speak. She had a severe stuttering disorder aggravated by adults around her failing to accept her as she was. She was, by her own confession, healed by a miracle after three decades.

I asked Trish if she expected to live very long, and she stated that she did not. She then related a heart warming story of her journey through letting go of her worldly possessions.

§

Trish. I am planning to move from where I now live to somewhere I like better. My son, John will help me move, but I am trying to work around his very busy schedule. But I have been packing and getting ready for the change in residences.

A very strangely spiritual thing happened to me while I was carefully dusting and packing my sacred religious statues, cards, relics, pictures, and books.

I became more and more at peace with knowing that I would not live very long. I found myself looking at my precious things and realizing that I might never see them again after I packed them away. But those things didn't seem to matter any more.

I became ever more aware that I would soon be seeing the very One that those things pointed me toward. The One in whom I have placed my faith, hope, and trust. Those aids to my faith would no longer be required, nor would they have significance in the presence of the Holy One they depicted.

This project became an adventure in letting go and moving on to something better. I was saying goodbye to the things of this present world and reaching out to the things of Heaven and my Lord. It was a wonderful, holy, sacred experience.

The things I had once held dear were fading from my heart and mind in exchange for things I now hold even more dearly.

The wonderful people of my parish church have prayed so hard for me, as I do for them. They are very precious to me. I feel their prayers and take strength from them. I attend mass at several different parishes in our diocese where everyone prays for me. Prayers and continually uplifting communications from them always lift my spirits. There is power in praying for others in intercessory prayer.

It has been my personal experience that the prayers of the sick are so very powerful with God. To embrace our crosses for love of Him the way He embraced His for the love of us is a prayer in itself. In a way, we surrender all.

I knew that there are medical breakthroughs every day in the field of cancer. There are also new types of cancer cropping up, new treatments, new hope, new technologies, and new research findings. That means that no one should ever give up or give in. We are all in this fight together.

I have gone through the hair loss, nausea, chills, mouth thrush, weakness, inability to support myself walking, diarrhea, and the rest. I have even been scared at times of what would happen to my body next. It is all a part of the protocol along with the waiting for the next report from the oncologist.

I remember each time when I went through a CAT scan; I knew Jesus was with me in that big tube and that He loved me. It was a very real love affair of the highest and most sacred kind. I would think, *'There is more of Him in me than there is cancer."*

I wanted to be thinking of Him while the machine was taking the pictures. I kept telling Him how much I loved Him, and I smiled the whole time.

I felt that if it was His permissive will for me to have cancer, how could it be wrong? And I knew in my heart that Jesus was more a part of me than was the cancer.

Through it all, I feel that I have become a better person because of cancer and the other periods of suffering in my life.

My faith is so much stronger; Jesus is so much more real. My prayers are more fervent and I am continually reaching toward Heaven and trying to become more of what God wants me to be.

I really would not change where I have been, what I have been, or what I have been through because of what I have become and am now. I'm so thankful; I love Him so much.

I tried very hard to detach myself from the things of this world and desired to be totally detached from earthly treasures and totally dedicated and attached to Jesus.

As I reach the end of my life, I want nothing to be holding me back, no encumbrances. I don't want to be found reaching back to grab something as I leave this earth.

Mike LaRiviere asked me if I knew what I would like my last words to be before I departed this life. I only had to think for a moment before answering him. I so desire that the last words from my lips would be sincerely uttered with a smile on my face. They would simply be, "Jesus and Mary; I love you."

Mike also asked me if I had any words of wisdom or advice to pass on to others. Yes I do.

Do not become attached to the things of this world, but seek to become attached to the things of the next world and eternity. Through suffering, especially cancer, we can become more at one with Christ who suffered so much for us.

There is a great deal of spiritual growth that comes through suffering and in no other way. I have been blessed through it all, and so can you be. One last thing; never, never, never give up.

As I readied myself to die from my cancer, I reached the point that I felt the need to simply hand my life and impending death over to my Lord and allow Him and my doctors to care for me. I had a peace that really did surpass my comprehension and I really thought I was on my way out of this world.

God has His own ways of helping us to grow spiritually toward Him and away from the things of this world. He is so close to us in our suffering.

My last trip to the oncologist reinforced my belief in God's power and love. My oncologist informed me that my cancer was gone and that I was cancer free. I would have a few more treatments to ensure the cancer was completely gone, but I had received a miracle. Doctors practice medicine and treat the many aspects of the disease, but only God heals.

§

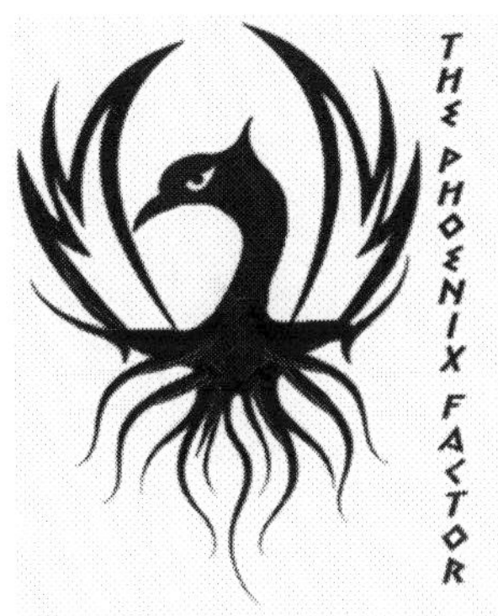

Mike. This has been a delightful account of the impossible becoming possible and that miracles still happen. God is very real, powerful, loving, and hears our prayers. Thank You Jesus, for Trish's miracle of healing.

I have tried to be careful in relating Trish's story without using terms, references, and theological points that might be confusing to readers who are not Catholics.

This is sometimes difficult to do, but I feel that anyone who suffers from cancer and the treatments that often worse than the disease will appreciate the power of faith, trust in God, the power of prayer, and the need for encouragement from others.

These truths transcend denominations and provide hope for anyone who calls on the name of Jesus in their distress. Trish is one of a precious few people who I find to be refreshing, powerful, uplifting, and absolutely solid in their beliefs. I simply could not let this beautiful story go untold.

§§§

Chapter Seventeen

Not My Baby! – The Strickland Family

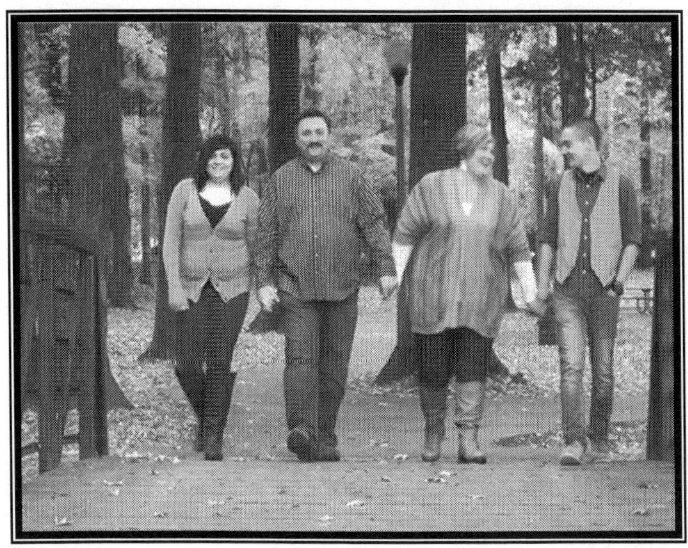

Pain, suffering, sickness and disease; death, grief, and mourning are all expected and accepted components of being a human being. They are the ever present threats that earmark being an adult. Even though they are unwanted, unwelcome, and mostly unplanned for, they usually come as no great surprise unless the disease is spelled ***heart*** or ***cancer.***

Heart disease, cancer, leukemia, diabetes, liver, kidney, and intestinal dysfunctions are growing and the older we become, the greater the chance that we'll suffer some type of serious malady. Someone once said "No one is going to get out of this world alive." That is a true statement, but we like to put off the inevitable as long as we can.

But, those are all things that we can expect as adults, usually older adults. We are supposed to die before our children and leave them to sort out our paperwork, estates and all the junk we have accumulated, and deal with our remains. That is the way it is supposed to be, and our minds, wills and emotions are geared toward that somewhat orderly scenario. But when it happens to our children –our babies, life turns upside down and things no longer make sense.

Judy and I wanted to include an account of how parents of a baby deal with the diagnosis of cancer in their precious young child. We found that case very close to home. In fact, this family is very close to our hearts.

Charles, Rena, Lynn, and C. J. make up the Strickland family. They live close by and C. J. just happens to be our future grand-son-in-law as it stands right now. These parents were faced with one of life's terrible truths that counter most of what we understand about diseases and flies in the face of the best efforts of parents to protect their children.

According to the American Cancer Society, the exact cause of most cases of childhood leukemia is not known. Most children with leukemia do not have any known risk factors, and from what is known, there is no known protection from it.

Even though science continues to study leukemia and all its parameters, there are very few known lifestyle-related or environmental causes of childhood leukemia, so it is important to know that in most cases there is nothing these children or their parents could have done to prevent these cancers.

We felt that the Strickland's had something significant to share with those who read this book. Lynn, the twenty year-old daughter can contribute valuable insights into our story in that she was the baby diagnosed with cancer (leukemia) and is now the young adult who beat the odds and won the battle with a fearful enemy, but lives in the shadow of a formidable disease.

I asked Rena about the early years of her twenty-one marriage to Charles that took place on July 10, 1993.

§

Rena. Charles and I worked at a grocery store where he was the manager and I worked in the meat department. As our interest in each other grew to affection and then to love, we knew that marriage was on the horizon and with that, I moved to another store that he didn't manage.

An immediate family was not in the plan, but God and human biology won out and I soon became pregnant with Lynn who was born July 6, 1994. We had our first, beautiful, healthy lively baby and the two of us became three.

At fifteen months old Lynn was stricken with a head cold complete with coughing, sneezing, and low grade fever. Her symptoms increased quickly to become what we thought might be upper respiratory infection and about midnight, she began gagging on phlegm. When her temp reached 102 degrees, we were off to Baptist East Hospital.

I knew in my gut that this was more than a cold and the quick advancement led me to believe it was more than an upper respiratory infection. The lab work at the hospital proved my suspicions right, but the results surpassed my suspicions in the seriousness of Lynn's condition.

Her white cell count was elevated and the doctor suspected viral meningitis that had been going around at that time. A spinal tap was conducted and when I returned to the room, I found Lynn to be covered with purplish patches or tiny red spots on the skin known as petechiae.

These tiny red or purple spots often appear in clusters, typically on the chest, back, face, or arms, and are a side effect of the blood's failure to clot. They may be confused with a rash, although they're really broken blood vessels and capillaries resulting from low platelet count.

Our pastor, my mother, Charles, and I were told collectively by the doctor at the emergency room that the symptoms and tests appeared to indicate Acute Lymphoblastic Leukemia, or ALL, or CANCER. We neither heard nor understood anything said after that.

Lynn and I were transported to Le Bonheur Children's Hospital by ambulance at two-o'clock a.m. Our family and pastor met us there where we slept, hung out together and just waited until we were sent to St. Jude's where we were admitted.

The next morning, Friday, October 13, 1995, the spinal tap was repeated and Lynn underwent a bone marrow test. Somewhere around lunch time, the doctor came in to inform us that our fifteen month old baby girl had leukemia.

Shock, trauma, and disaster impact people differently. But when they talk about your world stopping and graying out, time standing still, and emotions going into overload; they are all right.

Charles and I left Lynn at the hospital with family members, and we went home to gather our things for a stay at the hospital, the length of which was unknown.

When we entered our house without our baby, I felt myself losing it and I went into Lynn's room, dropped to the floor and melted into a pool of despair, despondency, confusion, and fear.

I don't know how long I cried or just what thoughts went through my mind. I do know the meaning of the term melt-down.

I battled with God, with my fears, frustrations, disappointments, and the fact that I did not want to accept the reality of what was happening. When I had exhausted my energy, resentments, anger, and confusion, I came to a point when I felt God's presence with me and I yielded my will to His. I said to him and myself, "Live or die, it's okay."

When we returned to the hospital we met terms like protocol, treatment, Hickman line, that is a central venous catheter most often used for the administration of chemotherapy or other medications, as well as for the withdrawal of blood for analysis.

We would learn about dehydration, platelets, white blood counts, hydration, IVs, side effects, and things to look for in a baby being treated for cancer.

For fifteen days we stood by while our baby was injected with chemo chemicals, watching while her tiny system was poisoned and observing every move that might indicate she was not responding well, or that she was succumbing to the ravishes of chemotherapy. Lynn went into remission after fifteen days, but continued weekly chemo treatments for 2 ½ years.

In the midst of her 2 ½ year treatment plan, We experienced another frightening side effect of medications when our toddler began having grand mal seizures from the high doses of methotrexate. Once when Charles was in the waiting room, he heard the call for the Harvey or Rapid Response Team and knew it was for his child.

Charles dropped to his knees and begged God to take him and leave his baby. This has become one of Lynn's favorite cancer stories, and it shows just what her father is made of.

Lynn was the poster girl for being a resilient child. She was one tough baby and played, smiled, and received everything thrown at her in good humor. A bit weak, totally bald from the chemo, some diarrhea, and monitored dehydration –but she beat the devil at his own game. Satan threw the worst he had at our baby, but our God stepped in and changed the rules.

On the last day of treatment, in April 1998, the doctor informed us that in only about one percent of the cases the patient responded as well as had Lynn. Remission came for our baby fifteen days after her first treatment.

Lynn would return for check-ups, tests, and monitoring once a month; then three months; six months; a year until she was eighteen years old.

That's how I saw it all. From a mother's perspective there is no fear like that which surrounds your baby who could die of a disease for which the treatment is often worse than the disease.

§

Mike. I have to break in here before Charles tells of his experience. I watched this family as they revisited the frightening aspects of the past and saw the reality of knowing that they all lived in the shadow of cancer now and in the future.

They cried during the interview, and I cried with them as their testimony brought back the spirits of my own experience to haunt my reveries. It made for a very honest, spiritually trying but uplifting interview.

§

Charles. Mike asked me about my feelings as I watched helplessly as my beloved was overcome with discomfort and concern. I couldn't fix the situation, I couldn't make it better.

This all came on the heels of my dad's death just days before Lynn was born. He was my hero and role model, and I wanted to be like him. He had all boys and Lynn would be the first girl in his family lineage.

We kidded back and forth about girls and he began to say happy things about her impending birth. He also had serious emphysema that would eventually take his life as he struggled for every breath.

I watched my hero die hard, and I blamed God for doing this to him and me. Why could God not let him live long enough to see his granddaughter? Why did he have to die so hard? He was a good man, a great father, and he was my friend.

As if losing my father wasn't enough, I'm now told my daughter has cancer. I became angry. I cried, I clenched my fists, I battled with God and I would have taken Him on in a fight as did Jacob when he wrestled with the Angel if I thought it would have done any good. I had a real problem with God over this, and it would take time to recover.

Being a father brings with it the faulty logic that you are responsible somehow for what goes wrong in your family and especially with your kids. I really felt helpless, somewhat guilty, and fully frustrated.

I have been in management roles for most of my working career and had many differing responsibilities. With each responsibility came the knowledge that if you applied sound logic, proven rules, and accepted management principles to any situation, you could expect somewhat positive results.

The situation with Lynn did not fit the mold. Cancer is not an exact science but involves abnormalities of human cells that respond to treatment differently with each person. A doctor can use the same protocol on one person who will experience remission. Another person may die of the same cancer with the same treatment.

PET Scans, MRI's, blood tests, and other monitoring systems and devices, stretched months apart indicate the success of treatment. The time between the test results is called waiting. The time just before each scan is called nerve wracking. The visit with the doctor to receive the results of the last scan is called a test and trial in positive or negative thinking.

§

Rena. When Lynn three years old, Charles and I found that we were pregnant again. Of course, we were concerned with our unborn child having leukemia and there wasn't much we could do to allay those fears.

At fourteen weeks, I went for a check-up. There was no discernable heart-beat and no fetal movement. An ultra-sound could not detect a heart-beat. The doctor suspected that the amniotic sac had collapsed and that the fetus was dead. A D&C (dilation and curettage) was ordered.

I hesitated and informed the doctor that I wanted to go home and think about everything. That's when my mother gave me a passage of Scripture from 2 Kings 4:14-37 that tells of a mother up in age that bore a son in a difficult situation under miraculous conditions. The boy later died, but was raised from the dead because of the mother's faith.

Our family fasted and prayed and our church family prayed fervently for us. When I returned to the doctor's office the following week, an ultra-sound found movement and a heartbeat. Our son, C.J was born healthy at nine pounds and fourteen ounces.

When C. J. started kindergarten, I went back to school and became a Medical Assistant and I work now at Baptist East Hospital.

§

Mike. It was interesting, challenging, heart rending and educational to listen to the Strickland's story. Both parents are sincere, honest, strong Christians and give God the glory for the miracles that surrounded both Lynn and C.J.

As I watched Lynn listen to the story unfolding, she wept frequently and I could tell she was sensitive to what was being said.

I explained to her that I wanted her to hear the entire story and then give me her side from a baby that could not understand the implications of childhood leukemia, through adolescence and the teenage years, and into young adulthood. She is now a 20 year-old young woman who lives in the shadow of the cancer she once had but is now cured. She shared some significant memories, trials, and fears that are worthy to be read.

§

Lynn. I guess that my emotions surrounding who I am, where I've been, and what lies ahead have come in large part from others around me. Their comments, my family relating things to me, and as I grew to understand what was going on, the doctors and care givers did their part in helping me to develop into the cancer survivor I am now.

I just have to trust my parents who were there as I was going through the chemotherapy ordeal. As a fifteen month-old baby, I remember nothing about it.

There was something about going in for checkups and tests that stuck with me for the first four and a half years after the last chemo infusion. I am not sure what being a normal child really means. Normal children don't get the kind or degree of attention I received. The attention was not always helpful, nor positive. I will never forget preparing for my visit to St. Jude's when I was seven years old.

I became apprehensive about the visit. Then fear swept over me as I began to contemplate with the mind of a child, the ramifications of who I was and what it was that had totally changed the course of my life. I adamantly refused to go for my check-up. I don't remember all that went in to convincing me to go, but I went.

I remember in school being called "that hospital kid," "radioactive kid," and other children would act like I was poison or dangerous because I had had leukemia. I tried hard to develop a thick skin and a hard protective shell. But that shell kept shattering and the thick skin wore thin quickly. Children are very good at being cruel.

I remember asking God, "Why me? What did I do to deserve this?" Months of crying, praying, arguing with God resulted in an answer that seemed very clear to me. God said, *"I gave you this life because you are strong enough to handle it."*

Then there were the abnormalities that occurred over the years. First, I developed a tumor like substance on my jawbone. The dentist called it a Neuroblastoma which is the most common extra cranial solid cancer in childhood and the most common cancer in infancy, and it turned out to be a bone cyst that we were able to have repaired.

Then there was the breast lump that turned out to be a non-malignant tumor. Then there was a benign tumor on my liver that has to be monitored.

I live on an emotional roller coaster where every new thing that can't be explained quickly becomes a major issue of concern. That's just the way it is with cancer survivors.

I heard a saying once that stuck with me and became my motto. "With Brave Wings She Flies." I am not a brave person so much in and of myself. But I turned it all over to my Lord along with my fears and He has made me brave.

As we were sharing our stories with Mike, I watched my dad weep at certain things and I wept also. Then Mike and my mom wept. My dad is my true hero, my shield and my protection. I love him with all my heart. His tears did not frighten me, but they allowed me to understand him more. He has a big heart.

§

Mike. In order to finalize the Strickland's story, Judy and I invited them for dinner and we had an enjoyable time of visiting and talking about family things. Each member shared their thoughts and present mind set concerning what happened nearly two decades ago, but still influenced their lives today.

Charles, Rena, Lynn and C.J. shared their faith, concerns, outlook, and hopes for the future. One issue that added a bit of emotion to the gathering was that C.J. the son, will soon be a United States Marine. If things remain as they are now, he will also become our grand-son-in-law when he marries our granddaughter, Scarlett. So Judy and I have a vested interest in the Strickland family.

I asked C.J. about his outlook for the future as he lives in the reality that his sister was at one time a very sick toddler and he had been pronounced dead in his mother's womb. I thought his response was mature, sound, and made me proud of this young man who had obviously been taught and parented well and paid attention to the preachers and teachers in his church.

C.J. said that he did not worry about contracting leukemia because it is not something that is normally passed down or around in a family. God had worked one miracle in his life by allowing him to be born and he has complete faith in Jesus. He also said something that gave me a lump in my throat. C.J. said that he was willing to suffer or die for his country if that is what he is called to do. This is Marine Corps material.

Lynn seems very well adjusted to not only her leukemia, but the physical scares she endured throughout her life. She stated that life gives us challenges and we can either run from them or learn from them. She once wrote how she felt about herself in a church meeting. She said "I am a survivor."

Lynn considers herself to be more aware of the world around her and knows that cancer is not biased in any way –anyone can get it. She is becoming more sensible and happy as she ages, and looks at her cancer as a change in the direction of her road of life.

§

Rena understands the medical ramifications of leukemia, protocols that deal with the disease, blessings of a place such as St. Jude's, wonders of living on this side of two miracles and gratitude she holds in her heart for what the Lord has done.

Their son has enlisted into the Marine Corps and will report for active duty when he finishes high school. This of course comes during a very troubled time in our world.

Rena is a praying woman. Still, in her mother's heart, she continually places her children in the Lord's care. A twinge of fear might come to her soul, and she finds herself visiting God's throne of grace and mercy. But she never loses heart or her confidence in God's love, mercy, and power of protection.

I saved Charles' story as the father for last. He will provide the Phoenix Factor. Of all the family members, I watched him during our conversation. There were times of deep contemplation, sometimes tears, sometimes looking up and away, and other times of manifesting the inner-most positive traits of being a father and husband.

§

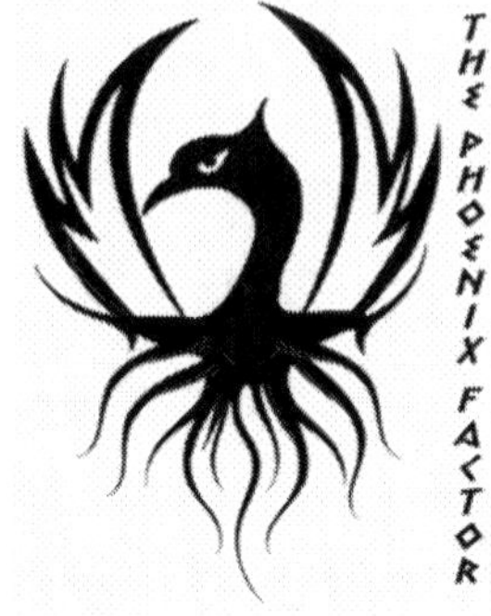

Charles. The picture that begins this chapter is of our family crossing a bridge at a local park. It's symbolic of three major events in our lives. We crossed one bridge when our daughter contracted leukemia and was miraculously healed by God with a lot of help by the doctors.

We crossed another bridge when we were told that our unborn son was dead and that Rena should have a Dilation and Curettage (D&C) procedure to remove the tissue from inside her uterus. Obviously, the doctor was wrong, or we experienced another miracle.

Another bridge awaits our family as our son C. J. as he is shipped off to boot camp with the United States Marine Corps and will leave his family and bride-to-be in order to place himself in harm's way for our country.

Our daughter was so brave and faced her physical challenges as courageously as I have ever seen anyone do so. Our son is brave and will face the calling of being a Marine with all the strength and heroism that is required. Their mother and I are proud of our children, and we feel that we have succeeded in rearing two Godly and capable kids.

§§§

Chapter Eighteen

Spark Plug – Pamela Genese Lockard-Freeman

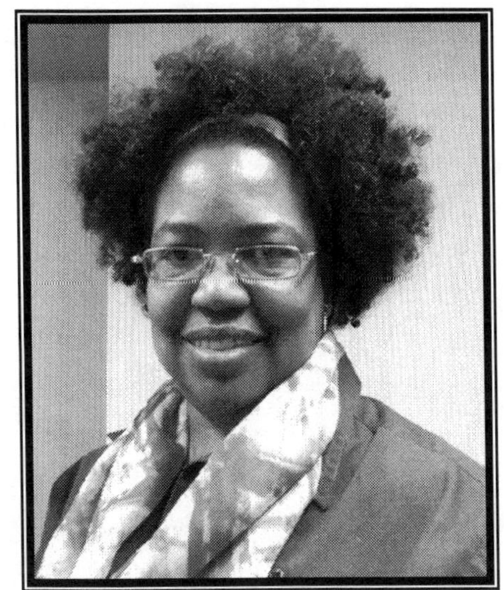

Mike: Judy and I first met Pamela at a Faith in the Face of Cancer support group meeting that is conducted monthly at West Clinic. Prior to actually meeting her, we heard about her from half the attendees as they introduced themselves and shared portions of their journey.

Pam's name was mentioned so often that it became comical. Many of the folks in attendance at each meeting were brought to their first meeting by Pam. If we were to create a Spark Plug Award for our group, Pam would win it hands down.

A spark plug ignites and is vital to the smooth operation of any gasoline powered engine. Pam is much like the spark plug in a vehicle; she gets it up and running and keeps it that way.

I have often said that there are two places where everyone is equal: at the cross and in cancer. Cancer is no respecter of race, creed, color, or gender.

Pam is a survivor of breast cancer for which she was diagnosed at the age of forty-five. She has had a variety of treatments after a lumpectomy, such as Mammosite Radiation and Chemotherapy, Aldriamycin, Cytoxan, Taxol, Herceptin.

This lovely, positive, articulate African American lady is married and at the present age of forty-nine is a veteran in the fight against this terrible disease.

We have already listed most of the side effects of cancer treatment, and we wanted Pam to concentrate on something a bit different than the woes of cancer, and tell of the strength in unity we have found in the togetherness of other survivors. We will now ask Pam to tell of her experience.

§

Pam: I was a strong, Bible believing, church-going Christian when I was diagnosed and that did not change during or after my treatments. The experience provided many opportunities for me to be obedient to God's will, to suffer for Him, as He suffered for me, and to depend upon His grace and mercy in my life. My greatest fear through it all was that I did not want to become disobedient to my Lord.

Mike asked me about my greatest disappointment. That would be that in my marriage my cancer experience didn't bring my husband and me closer to one another and my spouse didn't grow closer to God through it all.

I was also asked how Jesus helped me through it. I prayed to God for what I wanted and needed and he supplied me with ample grace, mercy and favor thru every step of my cancer journey. He provided support through my spouse, friends, coworkers and my church family.

God is so good. He granted one of the most important wishes; that I could continue to work during my treatment and not be sick from the chemotherapy. Hallelujah!

As of now, I am cancer-free. That is a term that every person diagnosed with cancer strives to hear from his or her oncologist. Some souls are blessed to receive a cure in this life while others will receive their healing in eternity. Why was I healed while others are not? I cannot answer that question; that rests with God.

§

Mike: We selected Pam to share her story in our book because of her strong faith, positive spirit, and her desire to reach out to others and bring them into the fold. Why would she do this? I asked her why she felt so strongly about Faith in the Face of Cancer, and she reinforced what I already suspected.

§

Pam: Our cancer support group is very uplifting for survivors and caregivers who are currently or who have shared the same kind of disease –cancer. It is facilitated by a minister who is our Chaplain, Sharon Herlihy. She is one of God's gifted and amazing women.

Sharon provides strength and encouragement to all of us. I find it a pleasure and a joy to be able to experience the group dynamics and shared experiences of every member. I gain much more than I give.

"My Mother, Mrs. LaVerne Lockard is eighty-one years old. God bless her; has been with me at every doctor's appointment, radiation treatment and every chemotherapy infusion. She attends the meetings with me and is a blessing to everyone she meets. I am most fortunate to have her in my corner.

Please let me share with you the Scriptures that have meant so much to me through my journey.

James 1:2. Consider it pure joy, my brothers and sisters, whenever you face trials of many kinds ...

Philippians 4:6. Do not be anxious about anything, but in every situation, by prayer and petition, with thanksgiving, present your requests to God.

Philippians 4:13. I can do all this through Christ who strengthens me.

Psalm 3:3. But you, LORD, are a shield around me, my glory, the One who lifts my head high.

I have chosen not to allow cancer and the subsequent brutality of the treatments to make me into a bitter person incapable of helping others or making a contribution to them in their journey.

In this troubled and hard world, there are many things that will destroy our witness to others and hurt our personal testimony about Jesus to others who need it.

I chose to rise above the disease, discomfort, distress, and devastation of cancer and to be an encourager to my fellow survivors. It has not always been easy, but through Jesus, it has been possible.

§

Mike: I want to break in here to say that when Judy and I first experienced the cancer support group, it was predominately African American, but I didn't notice that until later.

What we did notice was that there was fervent and animated prayer within the group. People were vocal about their faith, and they were sure about what Jesus was doing in their lives. I liked that and wanted more. That is what brought us back.

Amidst the powerful prayer and strong leadership of Sharon Herlihy, Judy and I found an oasis of spiritual refreshment in the desert and wastelands of this thing called cancer.

There were hugs, hand holding, eye contact, expressed love, and genuine sharing of concern for one another. I believe that the racism often associated with the Memphis area would disappear were it placed inside a family of folks such as our cancer support group.

I remember closing out one meeting and I broke out in a song; Thank you Lord for Saving my Soul. The next meeting, a strong and muscular African American man named Sonny came up to me and we both sang a hymn together. That brought the house down, and we both held each other tightly while we sang and afterwards. No- one wanted to depart after that meeting.

§

Pam: As I read Mike's comments, I have to confess that it is the power of unity, forgiveness, encouragement, oneness, and love that draws me to the group and prompts me to bring others into it. I have something wonderful to give others, and Jesus is at the center of it all.

Please allow me to share what I see when I attend a meeting on the second floor of the West Cancer Clinic Humphreys Center. If one will only open his or her eyes, he or she will see the same things as do I.

I see a recently widowed lady who went through a really tough time in the loss of her husband, but is spiraling upward in her grief. There is a truck driver, lonely and in need of friends.

A recently diagnosed sister having a very difficult time with treatment weeps freely. One person faces surgery, another is recovering from it. One reports being cancer free, while another is stage four pancreatic one week, and died two weeks later. Care givers come to gain strength for their life.

When someone calls out my name and smiles as she tells of my bringing her to the meeting, I feel warm all over. It's almost like bringing someone to Jesus, knowing it is the right thing to do.

I am so sold on the benefits of shared experience. My family is proud of me and so are my friends. And you know what? I am sort of proud of me also.

The list goes on, and for as many individuals as are present, there are that many unique stories and needs. Each one of us needs something, but each one can give something back. That is why I come.

§

Mike: Pam shared some of her favorite motivational Scriptures with me, so I thought it appropriate to share one of mine that contributed to our asking Pam to share her story.

Isaiah 61:1. *The Spirit of the Sovereign LORD is on me, because the LORD has anointed me to proclaim good news to the poor. He has sent me to bind up the brokenhearted, to proclaim freedom for the captives and release from darkness for the prisoners.*

To me, Pam represents the spirit of this passage. So many folks are broken hearted with the diagnosis of cancer either for themselves or a loved one. They become confused and often do not know how to proceed or what to do next.

I am always blessed by observing someone who cares enough to take a brother or sister in need by the hand and lead them to a place of rest and encouragement.

Care givers become frustrated over not being able to relieve their loved ones of the pain, suffering, discomforts and fears of cancer. Cancer patients often give up hope for a cure and resign themselves to a death sentence that may or may not be real.

We simply must be willing to take the essence of Scripture to these souls, and be prepared to give of ourselves to others in order to lighten their burden.

It is so refreshing for Judy and me to observe love in action; the Bible fleshed out in the lives of my brothers and sisters in Christ; and the reassurance that comes with a real life person telling others that there really is hope.

§

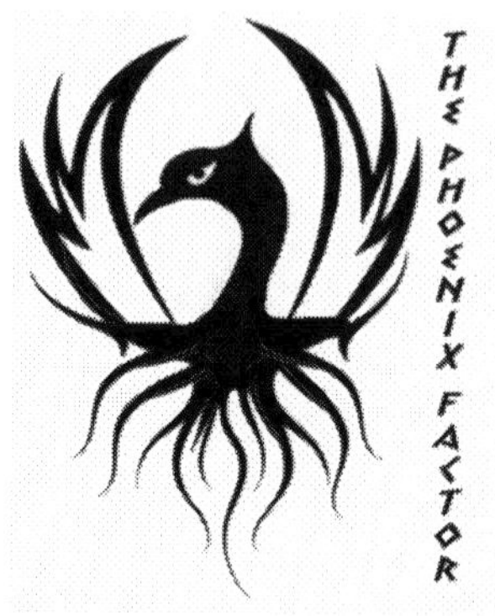

The apostle Andrew is known for bringing others to Jesus in the New Testament.

Pam is well known for bringing people into the Faith in the Face of Cancer support group and placing them in the care of the Holy Spirit.

She is quite a lady whom I am pleased to have met and now call friend.

§§§

Chapter Nineteen

The Afterlife – Living in the Shadow of Cancer

I attended a Lynn Eib seminar some time ago and came away feeling blessed, informed, and better equipped to facilitate a cancer support group.

I also feel more confident about assuring others who are diagnosed with the disease that there is life after cancer, and there are helps to living in the shadow of cancer. Lynn presented a segment on living in the shadow of cancer that I have drawn heavily upon in this chapter.

Definition of the term shadow: A shadow is an area where light from a source is obstructed by an object. It occupies all of the space behind an opaque object with light in front of it.

The cross-section of a shadow is a two-dimensional silhouette, or a reverse projection of the object blocking the light. Sunlight causes many objects to have shadows at certain times of the day. The angle of the sun, its apparent height in the sky causes a change in the length of shadows. Low-angles create longer shadows.

Shadows can impact us differently, dependent upon how we view them and just what projects the shadow. If a shadow is being projected from a helpful, friendly, positive source, it should make us more confident.

If a shadow is projected from a monster, a danger, a looming negative source, then seeing it will undoubtedly cause us concern or worry.

As cancer survivors daily live with the realization that they have either had or continue to have cancer, they can be bolstered in their journey in the fact that they move and live under the shadow of the Almighty, or they move and live under the shadow of cancer. It is a choice they will make for themselves.

Lynn suggested four verses of Scripture and we have quoted them from the New International Version of the Bible.

Psalm 91:1. He who dwells in the shelter of the Most High will rest in the shadow of the Almighty.

Psalm 36:7. How priceless is your unfailing love! Both high and low among men find refuge in the shadow of your wings.

Psalm 17:8. Keep me as the apple of your eye; hide me in the shadow of your wings

Psalm 63:7. Because you are my help, I sing in the shadow of your wings. My soul clings to you; your right hand upholds me.

The truth is that shadows cannot harm or help you, unless you are using them to shade yourself from the sun. Only the substance that produces the shadow can harm or help anyone. Your own shadow is just a projected image of the real you. By itself, it is harmless and can do nothing productive except provide evidence of the fact that you are close by.

If my granddaughters are present in my shadow, it is proof that I am near to protect and provide for them. It is the same with the protection promised and obviated in the Scriptures above. Of course, the shadow of a tree or structure can provide protection and relief from the blazing sun, and that is helpful.

One more thing; if we stare at the shadow of something frightening, we know that the substance of the shadow is lurking nearby. But the shadow of the almighty indicates that He is nearby and is always ready to help us.

Lynn said something else that stuck with me. She said that if we look directly into the sun, we can't see our shadow because it is behind us. The sun produces our shadow.

If we look away from the sun, we will see our shadow, but we will not see the sun. This is so true of keeping our focus on the Lord so that we do not focus on the shadows that have no real substance, but that do frighten us.

So it is with cancer. There will always be shadows that cause us to fear, remember, dread, and lose heart. The more we concentrate on the shadows, the more we will give in to the cancer that caused the shadows. Remember that what we see of cancer on the other side of remission is a shadow of what once was, but we fear could be again.

If the shadow is being produced by cancer not in remission but is terminal, it can steal our joy, cause us frustration, embitter us, and cause us to take our eyes off Jesus, who is the Hebrews 12:2 *author and finisher of our faith.*

Cancer survivors know firsthand about new pains, unusual body functions, and have all shared in the fact that the closer we get to scan days, the more symptoms crop up making us just know that the scans will show that cancer has returned or the tumor has grown.

§

Judy and I join countless thousands of cancer survivors who live on the other side of cancer. Treatments may be over, surgeries done, healing has taken place, we may be in total remission, and we are in the every two, three, six, or twelve month appointment cycle.

Some cancer survivors have lost organs, body parts, intestines, or have holes in their skulls, skin grafts, or have had vertebrae modified, marrow transplanted, or even organs replaced. These remind us of the cancer itself. But we are alive, functional, and still are present for our loved ones.

Some cancer survivors know full well the frailty of life and have no guarantee of tomorrow. Of course, none of us have that, do we?

§

To say that we are back to normal would not be true. The human body cannot go through what we have experienced and be the same as what it was before chemo, radiation, surgery, etc. But then, what is normal? I have alluded earlier to what I am about to say. But this is now my and Judy's *normal.*

Judy has lost a significant amount of her colon to surgery with subsequent chemotherapy, as well as having undergone a complete hysterectomy with her first cancer.

She lives everyday balancing certain foods, caffeine, dairy products, medications, and is faithfully involved in walking over two miles a day, five days a week. Failure to practice her disciplined regimen leads to nausea, diarrhea, dizziness, fatigue, constipation, and sleepless nights.

My life has changed significantly and the past year has suggested that what I am now is what I will be for years to come, if not for the remainder of my life on earth.

I have absolutely no taste or smell other than some sensitivity to sweet and salt. I cannot smell smoke, my shaving lotion, or even the occasional dead skunk along the road.

The major surgery I had in my sinus area modified that section of my face, but for the better. I now have fewer if any sinus infections, and breathe normally.

I cannot determine when I am full after eating, and so I am fighting a weight battle from the loss of 130 pounds during treatment.

I have only twelve remaining teeth; six in the front on top and six on the bottom. I eat much like a squirrel, but have no grinders and that poses its own set of issues.

My muscles are returning, but if I use my hands to do physically demanding work, my fingers and lower arms do the trigger thing and my muscles contract causing severe pain. I use muscle relaxer meds to ease the situation, or soak my arms and hands in hot water till the pain and contractions subside.

When I break a sweat or take a hot shower, I have the sensation of ants stinging me all over my body. I also have a cough reflex from the aftermath of the trach, and my voice has dropped almost an octave. I also have an obvious scar in my throat from the hole that was created for the trach.

I cannot allow my hair to grow out because it is growing from two directions and cannot be combed.

The portacath pulls on my heart if I move my arms a certain way and causes pain.

Now both of us have learned to live with all the above, and we are thankful to be alive. We are not complaining about these discomforts, we list them to suggest that whatever may become your lot after treatment, you can learn to live with it and then they become your normal. You can still be happy and have joy in the aftermath of cancer.

§

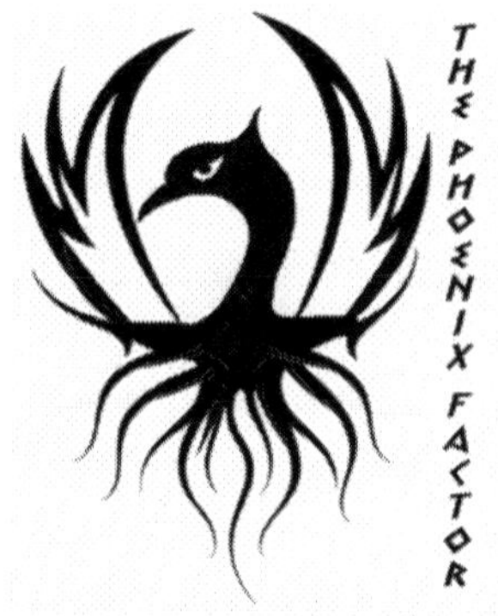

If we choose to live with the desire to have everything like it once was, we can become bitter and disappointed.

Wanting what we can't have is a sure way to become unhappy, dissatisfied, and lose our joy.

§§§

Chapter Twenty

Faith in the Face of Cancer Support Group

We mentioned earlier that Judy and I co-facilitate a cancer support group at Bartlett Hills Baptist Church in Bartlett, Tennessee, that is open to anyone at no charge.

We have undertaken this ministry in part due to the encouragement from and example set by WINGS Cancer Foundation Chaplain Sharon Herlihy.

It was under Reverend Herlihy's guidance, as we participated in the support group led be her, that we felt the call into this service ministry. She also assisted in providing the necessary resources for our group.

Our WINGS Cohort group is made up of cancer survivors and care givers who share their experiences and give mutual support and encouragement.

We laugh, we cry, we sometimes remain silent, and we pray. We are comrades; we are family. Our website can be viewed at

http://www.bartletthills.org/cancersupport.php

Judy and I worked diligently to put together the design, purpose, mission, and outreach of the group (actually it's a ministry). We felt that we had the makings of a sound program, but we also felt that something was missing.

We knew what our activities, agendas, resources, and focus would be, but we struggled with the overall design of the faith based endeavor.

We wanted to make sure that our personal best efforts were in keeping with Jesus' personal desires for His church and just what He would have us do in His name.

After we had put the proposal on paper, we submitted it to our pastor and staff for approval. We then went to our second home in Kimberling City, Missouri for a vacation and while there attended Sunday services at our church away from home, First Baptist Church of Kimberling City.

Pastor Jeff Hardy, who is himself a cancer survivor, preached a sermon we will never forget. He put into words and presented to the congregation of FBCKC the essence of that with which Judy and I had been struggling.

Pastor Hardy outlined what ministries of God's church should be about if they are to conform to His plan. In short, we walked away with the indelible impression that Jesus will build the church and we are to make and develop disciples. Amen!

According to the Bible, Jesus instructed his followers in the church, to go out into all the world and make disciples. That's what the local church is all about, or at least should be. We set out to be what we feel will help others and in doing so will make and grow disciples for Jesus.

In our case it's a matter of helping those who are usually already Christians to overcome a huge obstacle that has been placed in the path of their life and possibly spiritual growth.

Cancer is a disease of the flesh that can and often does impact the spirit and the maturing of one's spirit. As the old saying goes, "what doesn't make you bitter will make you better."

If you were to ask, "What is a disciple, by our standards?" We would say that "a disciple is someone who loves Jesus and wants to become like Him."

Since our group is a ministry of His church, we will do our best to help the members, who are already disciples for the most part, to grow to be more like Jesus.

It just so happens that our members have contracted cancer along the way, and can use some help and encouragement in that area so they can better serve the Lord as disciples and grow to become more like Him.

Among the most difficult lessons to accept and apply is when Jesus mentions *cross bearing,* such as in *Matthew 16:24-25.*
[24]*Then Jesus said to His disciples, "If anyone wishes to come after Me, he must deny himself, and take up his cross and follow Me.* [25]*"For whoever wishes to save his life will lose it; but whoever loses his life for My sake will find it."*

For those who are not Christians, we will show them the way, the truth, and the life. Hopefully, His love, reflected through our lives will cause them to want what we already have.

Cross bearing is about reflecting the person of Jesus Christ, His love, kindness, and mercy even in the process of dying and in suffering. Christians are to be gentle and loving even when we are in pain, or know that we are about to leave this world.

Christians, who have a genuine relationship to Jesus and have the assurance of their salvation, know that death is no longer the enemy.

The Bible assures us of our destiny and provides the promise of our personal victory through Jesus. *1 Corinthians 15:55* says, *Where, O death, is your victory? Where, O death, is your sting?*

The opportunity for Spiritual growth is greatest during these life issues that will come to everyone at some time or another. When we develop a healthy attitude toward both life and death, we can live in the freedom as the apostle Paul said "to live is Christ and to die is gain."

§

The church that God is building in the world has five points of emphasis for the ministries that belong to Jesus, but that He has placed in our care. They pertain to making and maturing disciples.

1. **Salvation.** Ensuring that everyone is pointed toward Jesus and that His love is reflected to each of them through us. This is of utmost significance in all that we do.

   Acts 4:12. Salvation is found in no one else, for there is no other name under heaven given to mankind by which we must be saved."

2. **Relationships/Fellowship.** Ensuring that each and every member is properly maintaining a meaningful

and beneficial relationship both vertically with God and horizontally with their brothers and sisters in Christ.

> *Colossians 3:12-17. [12]So, as those who have been chosen of God, holy and beloved, put on a heart of compassion, kindness, humility, gentleness and patience; [13]bearing with one another, and forgiving each other, whoever has a complaint against anyone; just as the Lord forgave you, so also should you. [14]Beyond all these things put on love, which is the perfect bond of unity. [15] Let the peace of Christ rule in your hearts, to which indeed you were called in one body; and be thankful. [16]Let the word of Christ richly dwell within you, with all wisdom teaching and admonishing one another with psalms and hymns and spiritual songs, singing with thankfulness in your hearts to God. [17]Whatever you do in word or deed, do all in the name of the Lord Jesus, giving thanks through Him to God the Father.*

3. **Equipping.** Ensuring that each person is provided with everything God has entrusted us with to help them to be what He wants them to become.

   > *Ephesians 4:12. to equip his people for works of service, so that the body of Christ may be built up.*

4. **Service.** Ensuring that each person is provided an opportunity to primarily use their spiritual gifts to serve other Christians and secondarily to serve others and bring them to a saving relationship with the Lord.

> *Hebrews 10:24-25.* [24]*and let us consider how to stimulate one another to love and good deeds,* [25]*not forsaking our own assembling together, as is the habit of some, but encouraging one another; and all the more as you see the day drawing near.*

5. **Replication.** Ensuring everyone has opportunities to replicate themselves in others and reflect God's love to a dark and dying world.

> *Matthew 28:19. Therefore go and make disciples of all nations, baptizing them in the name of the Father and of the Son and of the Holy Spirit.*

Making and developing disciples never ends and we are never fully developed in this life. We grow to become more like Jesus until we die.

It is a never-ending challenge. Like a five-pointed star, it takes all five points for the star to be balanced, symmetrical, and be what it was designed to be.

§

The concept we have just described is being taught and implemented at FBCKC and we are fortunate to have been present at its launch.

This approach is not revolutionary, but it does seem to answer the question that many churches are asking today: "Why are we here, and for what purpose?"

These ideas are not ours, they came from Pastor Jeff Hardy. Thanks Pastor Hardy, your inspired words will make a difference.

§

So you have it. Regardless of the pain, suffering, challenges, or opportunities we face, with a correct response, we will be able to face them and grow increasingly more like Jesus.

What would He do; how would He react; where would He go; when would He stop unconditionally loving us? If we truly desire to be like Him, those are what we would want to do. And we will not be content to do anything else.

§

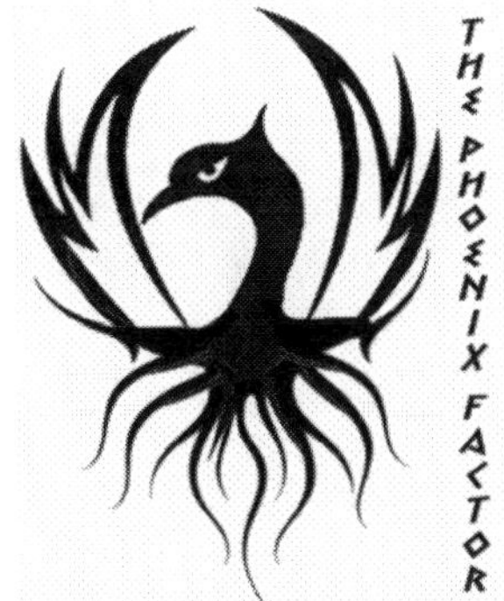

People today need examples of truth and what they believe lived out in everyday lives.

They look for others who are on-fire or passionate about their faith. These are things we try to bring to them in our support group.

Please allow me to say one very important thing about what I have already said. How we go about those six areas of focus must be done lovingly and almost invisibly on the surface.

Our members are there for support and encouragement. They will get all that, but it will be wrapped up in God's love and administered by His people, through His church.

When folks sense that what is being taught or preached is not sincere or does not pertain to them, they are hesitant to participate and they will not remain with the program.

Shared experience, love of God's people, a desire to help, and a willingness to be inconvenienced for others are all pre-requisites for being a contributing member of our group.

God bless you in your journey.

§§§

Chapter Twenty-One

A Tribute to Two Inspirational People – James and Renate Wood

In the early portion of our book, we made reference to Lynn Eib's When God & Cancer Meet, and how it has inspired us to write this book. As we close our work, we would be amiss not to mention two people who have inspired us to become who we are and much of what we have accomplished in our lives.

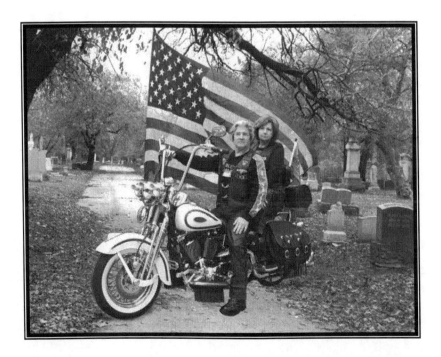

As we have said earlier, people today need real life examples of how to overcome tragedy and work through significant challenges in order to evolve into positive encouragers, productive contributors, and people who are at peace with themselves and with life. This does not mean that they are always happy with life or with what they have experienced.

Judy and I have been friends with Jimmy and Renate Wood for thirty years. Time, trajedy, trouble, danger, adventure, happy times, and hardships have molded us into best friends.

Jimmy and Renate are seasoned Bikers who ride a beautiful, chromed out, always clean and shiney (unless they are riding in the rain and mud), very big Harley Davidson Springer. They wear leathers, doorags, boots, and easily blend in with an Easy Rider motif. But don't let the looks fool you.

§

Let's travel back in time twenty-seven years. It's January 30, 1987 and I (Mike) am Jimmy and Renate's assigned church deacon. We were also friends.

The call that makes time stand still came informing them that Jason, their fourteen year old son had been critically injured in an automobile accident in which their first son, James Paul had been driving.

Jason was taken to Methodist Central Hospital where he remained on life support for a day. We had all gathered at the hospital, prayed, wept, held each other, and sat silently during the times when grief and sorrow took complete control.

A host of friends and family sent up great deal of prayers during that long and dreadful night.

Jason's head injuries were extensive and the family was soon informed that there were no indications of brain activity and that their loved one was not really alive.

This is ironic in a way in that many years before my late brother Frank was driving with me, five year-old Michael and three year-old Darrell in the car when we were broad-sided by a speeding vehicle.

Frank had just begun driving and he wanted to take us all for a ride in the car that Dad had purchased for him. He was so proud of that car.

Michael received the same injuries as did Jason Wood. Because he was so young he survived. He has a horshoe shaped scar on the side of his head as a souveneir.

I will never forget Jimmy begging me to ask God to send his son back. I had already prayed for that to no avail, and I explained to my friend that in my heart I believed that God had called Jason home to heaven and that he was gone.

I never want to do again what we then did. Jimmy and I walked arm in arm to the room where Jason was being maintained on life support equipment.

As we viewed Jason lying in that bed and not moving, we both prayed, and I sincerely felt in my soul the prompting of the Lord to stop the life support. We did.

§

I have watched this family go through grieving and mourning and parenting their oldest son and daughter through their own struggles.

I have personally seen heartbreak fleshed out and the ultimate loss overwhelm a family. I have watched as a mother resigned herself to a son dying before she did.

I was then, and have been, Jimmy and Renate's Sunday School Teacher for almost the entire time since Jason's death. I have watched the pain, the frustration, the confusion and loss spiral slowly upward producing the people they are now.

I think the hardest thing for me to watch was a father who helplessly stood by to watch the process by which his son departed this world.

Jimmy couldn't fix it, he couldn't stop it, he couldn't make the hurt go away. He was also limited in the comfort and relief he could provide for his beloved.

The greatest thing that I learned from this special couple was that an event such as Jason's death does not go away and you never forget it. You do learn to live with the pain and go on with life. That is something we can pass on to others who exerience a similar issue.

§

Let's go further back in time to about 1946. Renate Helga Braun-Dykierek was a very young child in Germany, who did not know her father. Her mother died at the age of twenty-three from dyptheria leaving Renate an orphan at six months of age.

She did not know until she was thirteen that she had been adopted by her uncle and aunt who were in their mid-forties at the time and who raised her in a strict but loving environment.

We need to understand that the private European social and family structure is a bit different than our American, open, tell-all norm. Many private and personal things were not discussed, confessed, or even referred to.

Things that might prove to be embarrassing or uncomfortable are simply not explored and are swept under the proverbial rug.

These memories still bless and burn. Renate's adoptive mom and dad are deceased and she seldom has personal communications with her few remaining contacts in Germany. Her family history and legacy still sometimes cause a bit of pain and angst as Renate asks the rhetorical question, "why?"

Jimmy was an Army soldier stationed in Germany when he met his Fräulein. They were married and they came to the United States, leaving what heritage Renate had in her home country. She and her charming accent came to this country and the two would make a life together.

§

Now it is June 3, 2014. The one man who I thought was impervious to most significant illnesses, went to the Veteran's Administration Hospital to undergo four heart bypasses during which he suffered a heart attack.

The surgery produced a Methicillin-resistant Staphylococcus aureus (MRSA) infection caused by a strain of staph bacteria that has become resistant to the antibiotics commonly used to treat ordinary staph infections.

A few other setbacks would leave him a bit shaky as he recovered over the ensuing four months. He has recovered and is almost back to what I call normal for my friend.

Jimmy is a lot like me in some ways. He was a career electrician, and as such he fell once from an elevated advertising sign and experienced significant injuries.

Motorcycle accidents have taken their toll, and retirement placed Jimmy and Renate in a fixed income situation that means less chrome for the Harley.

Renate fell and broke her back and she suffers from temporomandibular disorder (TMD) which occurs as a result of problems with her jaw joint (also called TMJ), and surrounding facial muscles.

She lives with pain nearly all the time. So that gives you a bit of their background. Why do we think their story is worthy to end out our book?

Nothing has been able to stop this couple from being wonderful parents, exceptional friends, outstanding Christians, and loyal supporters of our family. They are also unique contrinutors to our American way of life and society.

Jimmy and Renate are actively involved in a ministry to deceased military personnel, first responders, and their families.

Renate publishes on social media volumes of information in support of the Armed Forces and both are working members of an organization that was born out of ugliness, but is maintained out of patriotism and honor.

This ministry becomes more significant each day as anti-military and law enforcement sentiment grows in certain segments of society.

We are taking this opportunity to present to the readers the Patriot Guard Riders. We believe in what they do and are proud to honor their work and identify with them in this book.

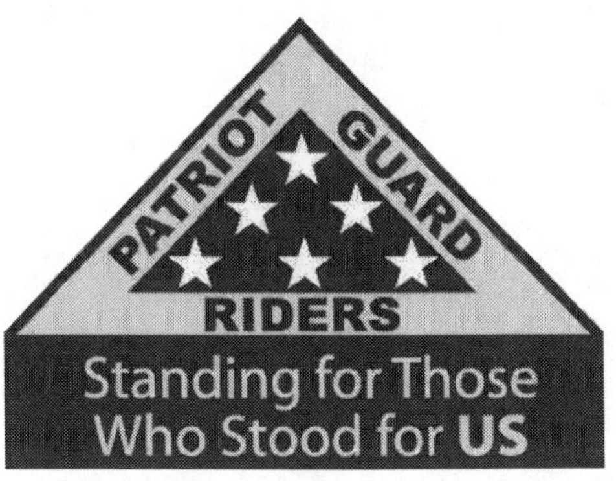
PATRIOT GUARD
RIDERS
Standing for Those
Who Stood for US

www.patriotguard.org

The Patriot Guard Riders organization is made up of bikers and non-bikers from across the nation. They are grounded in an unwavering respect for those who risk, or who have given their lives for America's freedom, way of life, and security.

It's not a requirement for membership that a member ride or own a motorcycle. Political views are immaterial regarding one's bend toward the right or left.

Members do not have to be veterans; it doesn't matter from where they hail or their income, church affiliation, profession, race, creed, or color. The only prerequisite is respect for the flag and those who have served under Old Glory or the public.

The PGR mission is to attend and stand at the funeral services and burial of fallen American heroes as invited guests of the family. Each mission has two basic objectives.

- First, PGR shows sincere respect for our fallen heroes, their families, and communities.
- Second, they shield the mourning family and their friends from interruptions created by single protestors or groups of protestors. This unfortunate and ugly situation is becoming more in vogue throughout our country.

PGR accomplishes its goals through strictly legal and non-violent means. Their presence is usually sufficient to quell trouble.

The PGR is there to back the men and women who are currently serving and fighting for the freedoms of others, at home and abroad or who serve as first responders to the public needs. They honor and support our military with every mission they carry out, and pray for a safe return home for all.

Through rain and stormy weather, sunshine, heat, and cold they ride in formation, carry flags, stand in formation along funeral routes, and stand guard at services in churches and funeral homes.

§

Jimmy and Renate have taken the hits life has inflicted upon them and risen like the mythical Phoenix to become a beautiful and powerful symbol of resilience and strength. They give to others and make a significant contribution to American life.

They stand and serve others in tears, in heartache, in discomfort, and many times in danger. What their life has been now has molded them into who they are and what they do.

I am always amazed and enormously impressed as I watch them minister while I know that in their hearts they carry grief and sadness that is often brought to the surface by that in which they are involved.

§

I want to close this chapter by mentioning the ultimate tribute that I have received by another human being. Let me tell you how really special they are and perhaps you'll also get an idea of just how unique they are and why they get a chapter of their own in our book.

Jimmy and Renate were on vacation in Branson, Missouri and were staying at the motel our son Michael managed at the time.

Late one afternoon, they received a phone call from Judy that I had been involved in a very bad motorcycle accident on our Harley and that I was in the trauma center of Saint Francis Hospital.

The doctors didn't know if I was going to live and the extent of my numerous severe injuries had not yet been determined.

Jimmy and Renate immediately packed, loaded their bike, and were on the road to Memphis as night began to fall with the bad weather that had moved in.

They had been up all day and had not yet slept. It would be a nine-hour trip in bad weather and road conditions, by two very tired riders.

Through high winds, blowing rain, mist, fog and splashing mud they barreled on through the dark. In retrospect, one biker to another, I am grateful that those loud pipes kept them awake.

I woke up sometime that night and saw two, muddy, wet, leather-clad angels standing by my hospital bed. I remained conscious only long enough to see them, but I remember that my heart leaped and at that time and I knew I would be okay. Sure enough, twenty some days later, I went home.

§

Judy, me, Jimmy, and Renate enjoy one of the strongest human ties possible. Jimmy and Renate are at the top of our list of heroes, colorful people, friends, and Christian brothers and sisters. They also ride a mean motorcycle and ride it very well; obviously better than I did.

Suffice it to say that if I need it and Jimmy has it, I've got it – and that goes both ways.

These two represent wonderful role models for recovery after life's worst black cloud has darkened one's sky. They really were and are black-leather-clad angels.

§

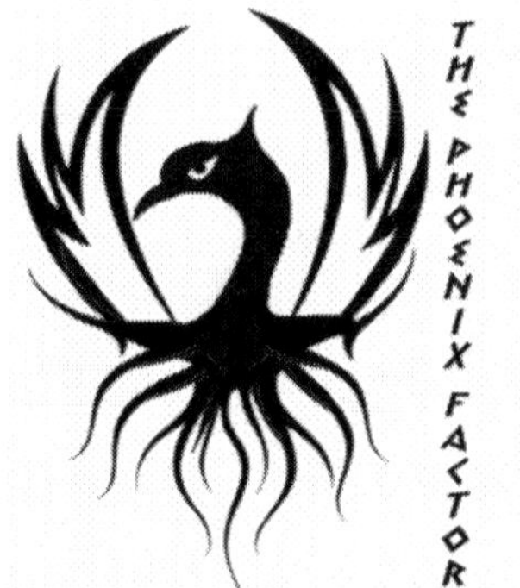

Hardships do not define character. Our response to the challenges of life do make us what we are.

As we overcome, survive, become the victors and are tempered in the crucible of life, we develop into who and what the world sees us as being.

The legacy that we leave behind will tell of how we responded to what we faced.

§§§

Chapter Twenty-Two

Learned Wisdom

In all of our dealings with doctors, hospitals, tests, follow-up appointments and the like, we have come away with a learned wisdom and intelligence when it comes to dealing with cancer. It would fit any disease, but this book is about cancer, and these insights relate to our experience.

Medical doctors have access to leading edge technology, research, established treatment protocols, and a highly skilled team of colleagues who stand ready to assist, counsel, and share experiences in any of the myriad physical abnormalities or diseases that might impact a specialist's area of expertise, such as ear, nose, and throat.

Briefly, they are trained to identify anything that is out of the ordinary in a patient's ear, nose, or throat physiology and the pathology that is involved in detection and treatment, such as was my case.

As specialists, they are among a group of physicians who normally see patients on referrals from other physicians; however, they also treat those who come into their offices on their own.

It is always unfortunate when physical anomalies have been left undetected too long and require what is commonly called heroic or emergency intervention to stop or hinder the advancement of cellular or immune system related diseases.

Often primary physicians and specialists with their associates become involved in treating patients late in the development of their symptoms requiring fast, significant, and possibly major surgery, radiation, chemotherapy, or other invasive actions.

When cancer is detected, a patient is immediately placed in the care of a Cancer Treatment Team to enter a tried and true protocol.

I came to my specialist through a referral from my primary care physician. I had a significantly formed tumor in my sinus cavity area and one at the base of my tongue.

As I have said, I was experiencing difficulty swallowing, breathing, and displayed numerous swollen lymph nodes around my neck area. I had complained to several physicians over two and a half years about these symptoms, but unfortunately, the cancer was not discovered.

When the symptoms became well developed and maturely proportioned, they were easier to detect and I was sent to an ENT group.

On my first visit, my doctor was able to show me on a computerized screen through the use of a lighted camera the two large tumors.

There was a real danger that the large tumor at the base of my tongue would swell when a biopsy was attempted and I would no longer be able to breathe. The doctor determined the need for a tracheostomy to allow an alternative breathing method prior to the required biopsies.

An MRI and biopsies substantiated his suspicion that I indeed had cancer and that it was Squamous cell carcinoma.

In reading this book, you have become well aware of the steps in my becoming cancer-free. In league with the medical team comprised of my primary ENT, an ENT advanced surgeon, neuro-surgeon, and oncologist they were able to achieve success in dealing with the cancer.

It has become my experience and studied opinion that patients who self-diagnose, or through apprehension of some form refuse to go to a specialist are begging for disaster.

Diseases such as cancer are tremendously invasive and exponentially spread faster than the body can deal with the out-of-control cell growth that earmarks cancer.

People, me included, will try anything to heal themselves of something that simply cannot be self-treated. It will eventually overwhelm the patient, who may be religiously eating, drinking, or otherwise consuming vitamins, juices, and products *guaranteed* to heal the body.

I did not, and still will not, accept a treatment program just because I am told I should do it. I research, ask questions, demand proof of need, and am not willing to put myself through unproven treatments and expect a good return on investment of anything the doctors treating me suggests be done.

I am open to discussion but often with arguments that must be satisfied prior to implementation of a plan. That is not necessarily a bad thing, as long as patients maintain an open mind.

I also made a critical mistake in refusing surgery to remove the residue of the cancer in my sinus. What I thought was a tumor no larger than an olive, turned out to cover half my sinus area, and the residue that was eventually removed was the size of a chicken egg, and was cancerous.

The surgical team was able to do extensive surgery and as

they say, “got it all.” I am cancer free, and I made some friends in the process.

§

Most of my dark journey involved my primary care oncologist. I learned a lot from him as well as the supporting personnel at the West Cancer Clinic.

Oncologists have a primary focus of identifying types of cancer, prescribing and monitoring treatments or protocols, adjusting medications, and intervening in the advancement or development of cancer in their patients.

Years of education, training, experience, and research position them daily to deal one-on-one with individual patients of varying ages, male and female, religious backgrounds, and those who may be terminal.

The specialist teams have access to the latest in technology, research, medications, and techniques that will ensure that each patient has the best possible chance of winning the battle with this formidable enemy called cancer.

Often, oncologists are incorporated into the treatment scenario of cancer patients late in the development of their cancer.

Either by denial, failure to address the symptoms with their primary care physician, fear of hearing the “C” word, or by self-diagnosing through information derived from the internet (which is normally inconclusive, in error, or written by non-professionals) they delay getting assistance from the professionals who actually can help them.

My oncologist was dedicated to establishing and maintaining a personal line of meaningful communication with me in which he encouraged openness, honesty, understanding, and firm yet kind two-way information transfer.

I felt confident that my doctor understood the frustration, fear, apprehension, and hesitation that I experienced as I dove head-first into a treatment system that proved to be brutal and uncomfortable. Openness ensured success where I believe strained, incomplete, or restrained discussions would have hindered the success of any protocol.

I researched and became well-informed, until I understood a great deal about physiology, limitations, and the dangers of any treatment such as chemotherapy and radiation.

I now admit that I was working under false assumptions concerning the Squamous cell carcinoma tumors that brought me to West Clinic as a referral from my Otolaryngology - Head and Neck Surgery physician.

Because of partial knowledge and misunderstanding the severity of the tumor masses and potential for recurrence, I was adamant about not having surgery to remove the tumor skin that remained in my sinus cavity after chemotherapy.

As I indicated earlier, a team effort of ENT, ENT Advanced Surgeon, Neuro Surgeon, and I convinced me of my error, and I authorized and received extensive but successful surgery.

My oncologist had the happy opportunity to inform both me and my wife Judy that I am now cancer-free. Had I not agreed to the counsel of five experts in my personal case, I am confident that my cancer would have returned very soon.

The field of cancer research, diagnosis, and treatment requires exacting knowledge and a continual application of diligent and continuing education to remain abreast with the demands and ever changing nature of cellular diseases. This is part of being an oncologist responsible for providing the very best care for the patients who place their trust and lives into their care.

My personal plea to anyone reading this book is "Please do not self-diagnose, instead, address symptoms with your doctor; do not let fear of the word *cancer* deter you from early intervention and probable remission or the extension of your life if you happen to have a terminal form of the disease."

I'll finish by saying that once cancer begins the process of developing in one's body, it probably will not stop. It spreads exponentially faster than the body's defense mechanisms can deal with the disease. You must get help and intervention.

The team at West Cancer Clinic will help you fight the battle with the best and most modern weapons.

My parting words to those reading this book are, "There are things that you cannot fix on your own. They are difficult enough to deal with when you have at your disposal the latest technology, techniques, medications, and research.

It is not wise to be your own doctor, even if you are a doctor. Let the experts work for you and you can expect to live longer and more comfortably when it is over.

§

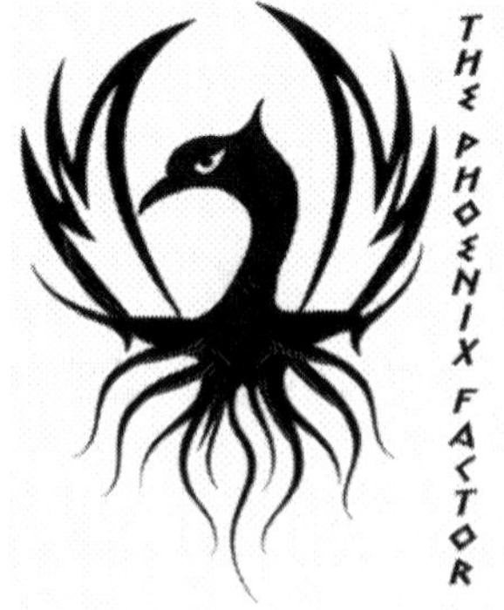

In my case, when I properly dealt with fear, denial, faulty information, and distrust of the very people who could help me, I was able to make sound decisions and avail myself of the resources at my disposal.

"What fools these mortal be."

§§§

Chapter Twenty-Three

Thoughts on the Scriptures used in Thank You God for Cancer.

We have provided a list of Scriptures that will be helpful if internalized and applied by cancer survivors and care givers. We have made a few comments only to get you started.

These can be a launching pad for a dynamic future. Commonly used Scripture with notes are from NIV Translation unless otherwise indicated

- **1 Corinthians 15:54-57.** 54When the perishable has been clothed with the imperishable, and the mortal with immortality, then the saying that is written will come true: "Death has been swallowed up in victory." 55"Where, O death, is your victory? Where, O death is your sting?" 56The sting of death is sin, and the power of sin is the law. 57But thanks be to God! He gives us the victory through our Lord Jesus Christ.
    - *If we are in Jesus, we have no fear of death, only the process of dying sometimes. We know what awaits us on the other side of that door –heaven and all things wonderful.*

- **2 Corinthians 1:6.** If we are distressed, it is for your comfort and salvation; if we are comforted, it is for your comfort, which produces in you patient endurance of the same sufferings we suffer.
    - *What we experience can produce good and valuable traits if we allow it. We also provide an example for our children and other Christians.*

- **2 Corinthians 12:7-10.** [7]or because of these surpassingly great revelations. Therefore, in order to keep me from becoming conceited, I was given a thorn in my flesh, a messenger of Satan, to torment me. [8]Three times I pleaded with the Lord to take it away from me. [9]But he said to me, "My grace is sufficient for you, for my power is made perfect in weakness." Therefore I will boast all the more gladly about my weaknesses, so that Christ's power may rest on me. [10]That is why, for Christ's sake, I delight in weaknesses, in insults, in hardships, in persecutions, in difficulties. For when I am weak, then I am strong.
    - *Pride, conceit, haughtiness, superiority, and egotism are traits that make it very difficult to do God's work.*
    - *When God empowers us to work through personal limitations, we realize His power and love and usually do not develop an attitude of being better than others.*

- **1 John 4:8.** Whoever does not love does not know God, because God is love.

- *Loving unconditionally, forgiving, and serving others must stem from God's love for us, or they will fail.*

- *Human love is often conditional and can run thin and then run out.*

- **1 Peter 5:6-10.** [6]Humble yourselves, therefore, under God's mighty hand, that he may lift you up in due time. [7]Cast all your anxiety on him because he cares for you. [8]Be alert and of sober mind. Your enemy the devil prowls around like a roaring lion looking for someone to devour. [9]Resist him, standing firm in the faith, because you know that the family of believers throughout the world is undergoing the same kind of sufferings. [10]And the God of all grace, who called you to his eternal glory in Christ, after you have suffered a little while, will himself restore you and make you strong, firm and steadfast.

    - *Cancer is of the flesh and the devil and from a corrupt and fallen world. There will be no cancer in Heaven and there will sure be no devil.*

    - *God knows and continually monitors our suffering in order to provide grace sufficient for our needs.*

- **1 Thessalonians 5:18.** Give thanks in all circumstances; for this is God's will for you in Christ Jesus.

    - *Can we really be grateful for cancer, pain, death, suffering of all kind? Yes, we can be grateful for our caregivers, doctors, nurses, and even chemotherapy and radiation.*

- **2 Timothy 1:12.** That is why I am suffering as I am. Yet this is no cause for shame, because I know whom I have believed, and am convinced that he is able to guard what I have entrusted to him until that day.
    - *God is in control, we are not. He is in control of our present condition and our future state.*
- **Acts 4:12.** Salvation is found in no one else, for there is no other name under heaven given to mankind by which we must be saved."
    - *Salvation is the heart and soul and foundation of everything else.*
- **Colossians 3:12-17.** [12]So, as those who have been chosen of God, holy and beloved, put on a heart of compassion, kindness, humility, gentleness and patience; [13]bearing with one another, and forgiving each other, whoever has a complaint against anyone; just as the Lord forgave you, so also should you. [14]Beyond all these things put on love, which is the perfect bond of unity. [15] Let the peace of Christ rule in your hearts, to which indeed you were called in one body; and be thankful. [16]Let the word of Christ richly dwell within you, with all wisdom teaching and admonishing one another with psalms and hymns and spiritual songs, singing with thankfulness in your hearts to God. [17]Whatever you do in word or deed, do all in the name of the Lord Jesus, giving thanks through Him to God the Father.
    - *Serving one another in the church is paramount to everything else alongside encouragement.*

- **Ephesians 2:14.** For He himself is our peace…
  - *Peace really is a person –His name is Jesus. To have a personal relationship with Jesus is to have peace.*
- **Ephesians 3:16-19.** [16]I pray that out of his glorious riches he may strengthen you with power through his Spirit in your inner being, [17]so that Christ may dwell in your hearts through faith. And I pray that you, being rooted and established in love, [18]may have power, together with all the Lord's holy people, to grasp how wide and long and high and deep is the love of Christ, [19]and to know this love that surpasses knowledge—that you may be filled to the measure of all the fullness of God.
  - *It is in the times of our greatest need and suffering that we are closest to God. It is on the other side of these that we can best articulate our gratitude to Him.*
- **Ephesians 4:12.** to equip his people for works of service, so that the body of Christ may be built up.
  - *The resources we have been provided in and through the Holy Spirit are to be used in the service of one another.*
- **Ephesians 6:10-18 (From the Message (MSG))** [10-12] …..God is strong, and He wants you strong. So take everything the Master has set out for you, well-made weapons of the best materials. And put them to use so

you will be able to stand up to everything the Devil throws your way. This is no afternoon athletic contest that we'll walk away from and forget about in a couple of hours. This is for keeps, a life-or-death fight to the finish against the Devil and all his angels. [13-18] Be prepared. You're up against far more than you can handle on your own. Take all the help you can get, every weapon God has issued, so that when it's all over but the shouting you'll still be on your feet. Truth, righteousness, peace, faith, and salvation are more than words. Learn how to apply them. You'll need them throughout your life. God's Word is an indispensable weapon. In the same way, prayer is essential in this ongoing warfare. Pray hard and long. Pray for your brothers and sisters. Keep your eyes open. Keep each other's spirits up so that no one falls behind or drops out.

- ○ *Life is hard and living a Godly life is impossible unless we avail ourselves of the resources God has provided. He provides power and comfort in our greatest needs.*

- **Exodus 15:26.** He said, "If you listen carefully to the LORD your God and do what is right in his eyes, if you pay attention to his commands and keep all his decrees, I will not bring on you any of the diseases I brought on the Egyptians, for I am the LORD, who heals you."

  - ○ *Even living in God's grace does not free us to sin and be involved in wrong living without expecting consequences.*

- *There are temporal and worldly consequences to any sin.*

- **Galatians 4:6.** Because you are his sons, God sent the Spirit of His Son into our hearts, the Spirit who calls out, "Abba, Father".

    - *This proved to be one of the most powerful helps to me.*

- **Galatians 5:22-26.** [22]But the fruit of the Spirit is love, joy, peace, forbearance, kindness, goodness, faithfulness, [23]gentleness and self-control. Against such things there is no law. [24]Those who belong to Christ Jesus have crucified the flesh with its passions and desires. [25]Since we live by the Spirit, let us keep in step with the Spirit. [26]Let us not become conceited, provoking and envying each other.

    - *People know us by how we act and treat others. If these traits are evident, people will know to whom we belong.*

- **Genesis 1:1.** In the beginning God created the heavens and the earth.

    - *God is the prime mover and maker of everything. He is fully capable of keeping it all running according to His plan.*

- **Hebrews 10:24-25.** [24]and let us consider how to stimulate one another to love and good deeds, [25]not forsaking our own assembling together, as is the habit of some, but encouraging one another; and all the more as you see the day drawing near.

  - *Mutual encouragement, respect, honor, and mercy will ensure harmony.*

- **Hebrews 12:2-3.** [2]fixing our eyes on Jesus, the pioneer and perfecter of faith, for the joy set before Him he endured the cross, scorning its shame, and sat down at the right hand of the throne of God. [3]Consider Him who endured such opposition from sinners so that you will not grow weary and lose heart.

  - *Jesus set the example for u;, He established our salvation; He maintains it, and He is the Guarantor of our covenant with the Father.*

- **Hebrews 13:2.** Do not forget to show hospitality to strangers, for by so doing some people have shown hospitality to angels without knowing it.

  - *We never really know who we serve or to whom we minister. We will, however, one day know.*

- **Isaiah 26:3.** You will keep in perfect peace those whose minds are steadfast, because they trust in you.

  - *No matter the turmoil, frustration, confusion, pain, discomfort or disappointment, you can have peace –even as we are dying. Trust Jesus.*

- **Isaiah 41:10.** So do not fear, for I am with you; do not be dismayed, for I am your God. I will strengthen you and help you; I will uphold you with my righteous right hand.

  - *God is for us and He calls the shots.*

- **Isaiah 43:1-2.** [1]But now, this is what the Lord says— he who created you, Jacob, he who formed you, Israel: "Do not fear, for I have redeemed you; I have summoned you by name; you are mine. [2]When you pass through the waters, I will be with you; and when you pass through the rivers, they will not sweep over you. When you walk through the fire, you will not be burned; the flames will not set you ablaze.
    - *Things may seem really tough, but God is always in control.*

- **Isaiah 61:1-3.** [1]The Spirit of the Sovereign LORD is on me, because the LORD has anointed me to proclaim good news to the poor. He has sent me to bind up the brokenhearted, to proclaim freedom for the captives and release from darkness for the prisoners, [2]to proclaim the year of the LORD's favor and the day of vengeance of our God, [3]to comfort all who mourn, and provide for those who grieve in Zion—to bestow on them a crown of beauty instead of ashes, the oil of joy instead of mourning, and a garment of praise instead of a spirit of despair. They will be called oaks of righteousness, a planting of the LORD for the display of his splendor.
    - *We are so powerful as we go out with God's anointing, in His power, with His instructions, and with His Gospel of Good News. We have such wonderful gifts to bestow, such peace, such comfort.*

- **James 1:2**. Consider it pure joy, my brothers and sisters, whenever you face trials of many kinds …

- *We will become better or bitter whatever may befall us.*

- **James 1:12.** Blessed is the one who perseveres under trial because, having stood the test, that person will receive the crown of life that the Lord has promised to those who love him.

  - *God sees and allows everything that happens to us and he is the judge of our performance and response.*

- **Jeremiah 29:11–13.** [11]For I know the plans I have for you," declares the LORD, "plans to prosper you and not to harm you, plans to give you hope and a future. [12]Then you will call on me and come and pray to me, and I will listen to you. [13]You will seek me and find me when you seek me with all your heart.

  - *If it is of God, it is for our good.*

- **John 6:35.** Then Jesus declared, "I am the bread of life. Whoever comes to me will never go hungry, and whoever believes in me will never be thirsty."

  - *Jesus is the provider of all that we need.*

- **John 11:25-26.** [25]Jesus said to her, "I am the resurrection and the life. The one who believes in me will live, even though they die; [26]and whoever lives by believing in me will never die. Do you believe this?"
  - *Do you believe this? That may be the only promise remaining for some cancer sufferers.*

- **John 14:6.** Jesus answered, "I am the way and the truth and the life. No one comes to the Father except through me."
    - *There is no other way to salvation or truth.*

- **John 14:26.** But the Advocate, the Holy Spirit whom the Father will send in my name will teach you all things and will remind you of everything I have said to you.
    - *We have the indwelling Holy Spirit to guide us in our lives.*

- **John 14:27.** Peace I leave with you; my peace I give you. I do not give to you as the world gives. Do not let your hearts be troubled and do not be afraid.
    - *We have peace in whatever state we are in. We may not avail ourselves of it, but it is there.*

- **John 16:33.** I have told you these things, so that in me you may have peace. In this world you will have trouble. But take heart! I have overcome the world.
    - *Nothing can happen to us over which God does not have control.*

- **Luke 9:23.** *"Then he said to them all: "Whoever wants to be my disciple must deny themselves and take up their cross daily and follow me."*
    - *Cross bearing has to do with suffering, pain, death, discomfort and other opportunities to share in Christ's suffering and death for us.*

- **Mark 11:24.** Therefore I tell you whatever you ask for in prayer believe that you have received it, and it will be yours.
    - *This is not carte-blanche for things not in God's will.*
- **Mark 12:31.** The second is this: "Love your neighbor as yourself." There is no commandment greater than these."
    - *Love for our fellow man motivates us to do most of what we do in ministry –or the lack of it.*
- **Matthew 11:28-29.** [28]Come to me, all you who are weary and burdened, and I will give you rest. [29]Take my yoke upon you and learn from me, for I am gentle and humble in heart, and you will find rest for your souls.
    - *There will be times when people on the journey will become exhausted and totally spent. Jesus has promised to provide rejuvenation when we need it most.*
- **Matthew 16:24-25.** [24]Then Jesus said to His disciples, "If anyone wishes to come after Me, he must deny himself, and take up his cross and follow Me. [25]"For whoever wishes to save his life will lose it; but whoever loses his life for My sake will find it. For those who are not Christians, we will show them the way, the truth, and the life. Hopefully, His love, reflected through our lives will cause them to want what we already have.
    - *Being kind and considerate of others while we ourselves are in pain or in the process of dying is true spiritual maturity.*

- **Matthew 28:19.** Therefore go and make disciples of all nations, baptizing them in the name of the Father and of the Son and of the Holy Spirit.
    - *The only way the church will grow and thrive is by the replicating ourselves as disciples.*
- **Philippians 3:7-10.** [7]But whatever were gains to me I now consider loss for the sake of Christ. [8]What is more, I consider everything a loss because of the surpassing worth of knowing Christ Jesus my Lord, for whose sake I have lost all things. I consider them garbage, that I may gain Christ [9]and be found in him, not having a righteousness of my own that comes from the law, but that which is through faith in Christ—the righteousness that comes from God on the basis of faith. [10]I want to know Christ—yes, to know the power of his resurrection and participation in his sufferings, becoming like him in his death, [11]and so, somehow, attaining to the resurrection from the dead.
    - *The more we become like Jesus, the less worldly things will matter.*
- **Philippians 4:6-7.** [6]Do not be anxious about anything, but in every situation, by prayer and petition, with thanksgiving, present your requests to God. [7]And the peace of God, which transcends all understanding, will guard your hearts and your minds in Christ Jesus.
    - *Being held in Abba, Daddy's arms, feeling His presence, totally collapsing into His care, that peace cannot be explained, but it sure can be felt.*

- **Philippians 4:8.** Finally, brothers and sisters, whatever is true, whatever is noble, whatever is right, whatever is pure, whatever is lovely, whatever is admirable —if anything is excellent or praiseworthy —think about such things.
    - *Think positive, pure, and precious thoughts. They are filled with power and light.*
- **Philippians 4:11-13.** [11]I am not saying this because I am in need, for I have learned to be content whatever the circumstances. [12]I know what it is to be in need, and I know what it is to have plenty. I have learned the secret of being content in any and every situation, whether well fed or hungry, whether living in plenty or in want. [13]I can do all this through him who gives me strength.
    - *Scripture does not say our lot will be easy or even fast. Be patient, be still and listen to His still small voice; rest in Him.*
    - *Not necessarily quickly or easily, but all things within God's will can be done through Christ.*
- **Psalm 3:3.** But you, LORD, are a shield around me, my glory, the One who lifts my head high.
    - *He is our protection, our provision, our strength and our reward.*
- **Psalm 17:8.** Keep me as the apple of your eye; hide me in the shadow of your wings.
    - *We are very special to God.*

- **Psalm 22:1-2.** [1]My God, my God, why have you forsaken me? Why are you so far from saving me, so far from my cries of anguish? [2]My God, I cry out by day, but you do not answer, by night, but I find no rest.
    - *There will be times when, like in David's case, we think God does not hear or care. We would be wrong.*

- **Psalm 23.** [1]The LORD is my shepherd, I lack nothing. [2]He makes me lie down in green pastures, he leads me beside quiet waters, [3]he refreshes my soul. He guides me along the right paths for his name's sake. [4]Even though I walk through the darkest valley, I will fear no evil, for you are with me; your rod and your staff, they comfort me. [5]You prepare a table before me in the presence of my enemies. You anoint my head with oil; my cup overflows. [6]Surely your goodness and love will follow me all the days of my life, and I will dwell in the house of the LORD forever.
    - *This Psalm stands out as one of our favorite comfort and assurance Scriptures. I have said it dozens of times. It is beautiful, powerful, and transforming.*

- **Psalm 28:7.** The LORD is my strength and my shield; my heart trusts in him, and he helps me. My heart leaps for joy, and with my song I praise him.
    - *Jesus is the all-in-all for the Christian.*

- **Psalm 29:11.** The LORD gives strength to his people; the LORD blesses his people with peace.

  - *We can always experience peace in the midst of a storm tossed life and be strong in the bond of weakness.*

- **Psalm 30:5.** [5b]Weeping may stay for the night, but rejoicing comes in the morning.

  - *There will be times in the night when we will pray earnestly for the morning to come.*

- **Psalm 36:7.** How priceless is your unfailing love O God! People take refuge in the shadow of your wings.

  - *God loves all men unconditionally.*

- **Psalm 46:1-2.** [1]God is our refuge and strength, an ever-present help in trouble. [2]Therefore we will not fear, though the earth give way and the mountains fall into the heart of the sea.

  - *Because we belong to God, nothing can destroy our security unless we allow it.*

- **Psalm 50:15. ...**and call on me in the day of trouble; I will deliver you, and you will honor me.

  - *Sometimes by healing, sometimes long term suffering, sometimes death and home-going. You will be delivered.*

- **Psalm 63:7-8.** [7]Because you are my help, I sing in the shadow of your wings. [8]I cling to you; your right hand upholds me.

- *Like when we were just kids and we stood by our earthly father's side. We could whip the world.*

- **Psalm 69:1-3.** [1]Save me, O God, for the waters have come up to my neck. [2]I sink in the miry depths, where there is no foothold. I have come into the deep waters; the floods engulf me. [3]I am worn out calling for help; my throat is parched. My eyes fail, looking for my God.
  - *If we are honest, we all have felt that God doesn't hear us at times. It does not mean that He does not hear us, it usually means that He is allowing us to be further prepared for His answer.*

- **Psalm 77:14.** You are the God who performs miracles; You display Your power among the peoples.
  - *God did and still does work miracles for his people.*

- **Psalm 91:1-4.** [1]Whoever dwells in the shelter of the Most High will rest in the shadow of the Almighty. [2]I will say of the LORD, "He is my refuge and my fortress, my God, in whom I trust." [3]Surely he will save you from the fowler's snare and from the deadly pestilence. [4]He will cover you with his feathers, and under his wings you will find refuge; his faithfulness will be your shield and rampart (buckler).
  - *As husbands protect their families, God protects his children even more so.*

- **Psalm 116:1.** I love the LORD, for He heard my voice; He heard my cry for mercy. Because He turned His ear to me, I will call on Him as long as I live.

- *The Lord sees and hears an knows our state even before we tell Him.*

- **Psalm 138:8.** The Lord will vindicate me; Your love Lord endures forever, do not abandon the work of your hands.

  - *God is not finished with us yet, far from it. But He will finish what He started.*

- **Psalm 139:1-4.** [1]You have searched me, LORD, and you know me. [2]You know when I sit and when I rise; you perceive my thoughts from afar. [3]You discern my going out and my lying down; you are familiar with all my ways. [4]Before a word is on my tongue you, LORD, know it completely.

  - *God already knows how sick we are, how we hurt, what we fear, that we are out of control. He has already gone before us to prepare the way. He didn't give us cancer, but He is in it with us.*

- **Revelation 21:4-5**. [4]He will wipe every tear from their eyes. There will be no more death or mourning or crying or pain, for the old order of things has passed away. [5]He who was seated on the throne said, "I am making everything new!" Then he said, "Write this down, for these words are trustworthy and true."

  - *When I lay dying, feeling my life ebb away, seeing all around me fade into oblivion, I waited the Death Angel's appearance. Peace came, freedom from care, and I fully resigned to the wonder of the transition from this life to the next. I really looked forward to it. Then I woke up in the hospital.*

- **Revelation 22:13.** I am the Alpha and the Omega, the First and the Last, the Beginning and the End.
    - *God is all in all and is outside the parameters of everything that is. He is greater than His creation and more powerful than all the energy of the universe,*
- **Romans 1:7.** To all in Rome who are loved by God and called to be his holy people: Grace and peace to you from God our Father and from the Lord Jesus Christ.
    - *Everything man-ward from God is called grace. We are the object of His mercy, grace, love, and peace.*
- **Romans 5:3-4.** [3]… but we also glory in our sufferings, because we know that suffering produces perseverance; [4]perseverance, character; and character, hope.
    - *There is nothing on earth to compare with the wonders of what He has in store for those who take up their cross and follow Him in suffering and even death.*
- **Romans 8:15**, The Spirit you received does not make you slaves, so that you live in fear again; rather, the Spirit you received brought about your adoption to sonship. And by him we cry, "Abba, Father."
    - *Not a slave but a son. Almighty God is my Father.*

- **Romans 8:18.** I consider that our present sufferings are not worth comparing with the glory that will be revealed in us.
    - *Sometimes promises of Scripture are hard to grasp because we go through difficulties so hard to accept as paling in the light of promise.*

- **Romans 8:22-25.** [22]We know that the whole creation has been groaning as in the pains of childbirth right up to the present time. [23]Not only so, but we ourselves, who have the first fruits of the Spirit, groan inwardly as we wait eagerly for our adoption to sonship, the redemption of our bodies. [24]For in this hope we were saved. But hope that is seen is no hope at all. Who hopes for what they already have? [25]But if we hope for what we do not yet have, we wait for it patiently.
    - *This is not all there is, the best is yet to come.*

- **Romans 8:26-27.** [26]In the same way, the Spirit helps us in our weakness. We do not know what we ought to pray for, but the Spirit himself intercedes for us through wordless groans. [27]And he who searches our hearts knows the mind of the Spirit, because the Spirit intercedes for God's people in accordance with the will of God.
    - *When we cannot even voice our need, when we are totally overwhelmed to the point of silence, or if we have totally surrendered to the disease, the Holy Spirit, who lives in us, prays for us, better than we can do for ourselves.*

- **Romans 8:28.** And we know that in all things God works for the good of those who love him, who have been called according to his purpose.
    - *Even if our cancer is unto death, God can bring good from it, usually in the form of spiritual growth and maturity for us and others.*
- **Romans 12:2.** Do not conform to the pattern of this world, but be transformed by the renewing of your mind. Then you will be able to test and approve what God's will is--his good, pleasing and perfect will.
    - *God's ways are much different than are those of the world. Sometimes they are opposite of what the world accepts as normal.*
- **Romans 15:13.** [13]May the God of hope fill you with all joy and peace as you trust in him, so that you may overflow with hope by the power of the Holy Spirit.
    - *You can be filled with hope and glory and in being so find that your salvation and being kept by the Holy Spirit will be effervescent and bubbling over.*
- **Zephaniah 3:17**. The Lord your God is with you, the Mighty Warrior who saves. He will take great delight in you; in His love, He will no longer rebuke you but will rejoice over you with singing.
    - *The Father loves us like His Son Jesus and both take pride in us. The Father, Son and Holy Spirit are one and as one think we are very special.*

§

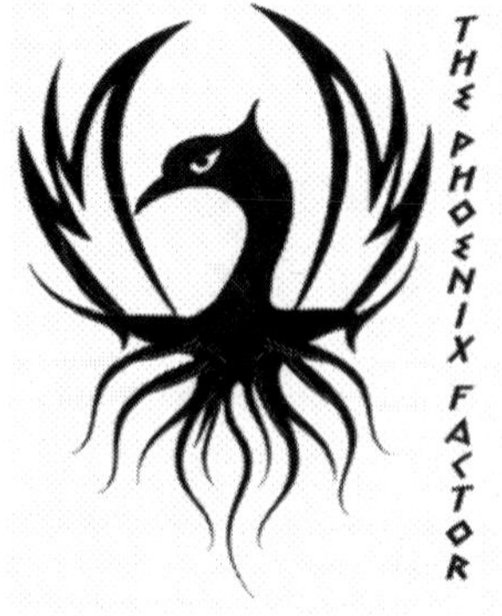

The Phoenix Factor for each chapter of Thank You God for Cancer relates to the precious promises, comfort, encouragement, and power of what God has provided in Scripture.

As bad as cancer can be, the victory is sweeter. As harsh as the treatments can be the peace and assurance of Scripture makes it bearable and through that assurance, we can see light at the end of the tunnel and a bright future either here in this life or with Jesus in eternity.

§§§

Other Books by the Author

1. **Eden's Door – The Beginning**
A trip back through history to the time of Jesus

2. **Eden's Door – Hell's Gate**
When present day meets a bygone era and man meets demon

3. **Demon Rising**
History culminates with the rapture as the physical joins the metaphysical and spirits interact with men

4. **Indian Summer – The Last Pow Wow**
A Native American heritage comes alive

5. **The Last Pow Wow – Death of a Spirit**
Making the most of a rich Native American heritage

6. **The Christmas Box** – with Judy LaRiviere
Leaving a legacy through gift giving

7. **Black Clouds and Little Angels**
The story of our son's struggles and victories

8. **The Tale of Brown Horsey – A Children's Book**
Illustrated dreamscape of our granddaughter's favorite plush animals coming to life
(Not available through Amazon.com)

9. **FantasyLand – A Children's Novel**
Illustrated journey of our granddaughters to and from a fantasy world populated with familiar faces

10. **Snake Oil – An Enoch Hardy Mystery**
with D E LaRiviere
A small town sheriff fights crime while maintaining a strong Christian character

11. **Dark Rider – An Enoch Hardy Mystery**
A mysterious stranger with unusual insights and powers comes to town and helps the sheriff deal with a situation way over his head

12. **Rampage – An Enoch Hardy Mystery**
A storm, a broken dam, and a flood overwhelm the sheriff's town and countryside as serial criminals wreak havoc on innocent people

13. **Hidden – An Enoch Hardy Mystery**
A terrorist threat so significant as to require a counterforce of the law and the lawless to join in an effort to stop it

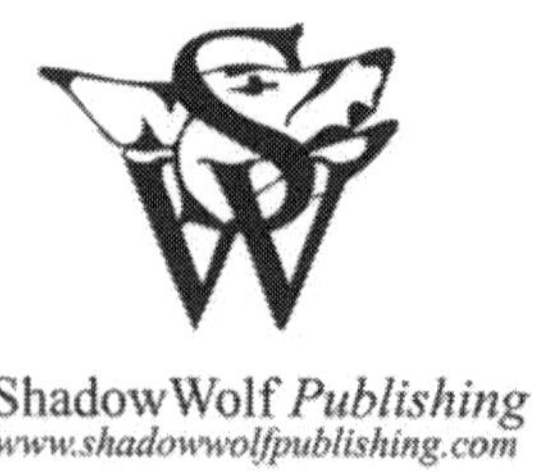

ShadowWolf *Publishing*
www.shadowwolfpublishing.com

All books are available through Amazon.com

Made in the USA
Lexington, KY
10 August 2015